RESISTANCE TRAINING: FOR MARTIAL ARTIST, MIXED MARTIAL ARTS (MMA), BOXING AND ALL COMBAT FIGHTS

Resistance Training: For Martial Artist, Mixed Martial Arts (MMA), Boxing and All Combat Fights

G. E. S. BOLEY, JR., MBA, CFT, CSN

CONTENTS

AUTHOR'S NOTES

The purpose of this book is to put a creditable training manual in place that is built around the basics of resistance training. In short, this book compiles proven training principles I use to teach my clients and students, with the latest basic weight training routines. Far too often, people get caught up in the *"new and improved"* craze at their gym, forgetting about basic movements and training principles. I hope that my efforts help you to reach your training goals.

G. E. S. Boley, Jr. MBA, CTF, CSN

I would personally like to thank my family for keeping me focused on what's important. Including my cousin Mr. Kenneth "Tiny" Glover (RIP), for being my first personal trainer (at the age of 14), and teaching me how to train properly and drug-free! My parents for enrolling me in martial arts classes at such a young age. My wife and kids for being my support system when the world wasn't! Included in these thanks are my Grandmaster (Instructor) Mr. Robert N. Wheatley for asking me to put my experiences on paper and Master Nick Malefyt for being a great instructor, friend, and brother, not only in martial arts but in life, and for picking me up when I was in a low place. Lastly, I would also like to thank everybody who believed in me and shared their vast knowledge with me.

INTRODUCTION

Remember: As always, before you start any training regimen or taking any supplements, consult your physician first! Also, remember when weight lifting, "at all times, you control the weight and muscle movements. The weight should never be controlling you!" If this happens, then you should adjust the weight to a manageable amount, or, start the movements with NO weight at all!

One good technique is to practice a lift with just a weight bar until you have the move under control. Then add weights.

Did you know that more than 50% of all gym memberships go unused? Most people, actually 90%, quit working out within the first three months of starting a gym membership. There is a nationwide lack of obtainable expectations and realistic fitness goals. Most people suffer from a lack of motivation. It is cool in the beginning but, like everything else, once that new burst of excitement is gone, it is really hard to stay focused. You need that motivation to get through a plateau. To push through a barrier when your body stops responding like it previously did.

This is when most people quit. Or do something else.

Far too many times, I see beginners walk into a gym and just do

EVERYTHING! No focus. No idea what they are trying to accomplish and no pathway to get them there. They take the 40-minute introduction the gym gave them on the machines and weights and do that same workout every time they come in. How can you get anything accomplished when you really don't know what you are doing? It's more than likely this cycle of training that causes the high dropout rate on those memberships.

Young members then start looking at other sources for tips and ideas - like online videos and magazines - for routines that don't have any real substance to them but are great "eye candy". So when they try that routine or lift that load they saw in the video, they can't do it. Or worse, they push it to the point where they lift the weight, like in bench pressing, but the technique is wrong. Their back is arched and off the bench in terrible form, they don't let the weight go all the way down to the brim of the chest or their feet are off the ground, and they injure themselves. I HATE seeing members accomplish the lift with that bad technique because they have a (false) mental accomplishment that ultimately kills their chances of long-term fitness success and ten times out of ten results in injury! This can happen with any body part when training as an unknowledgeable beginner.

But after 32 years, I found that resistance training is rarely about lifting huge weights. Basic resistance training can include such things as raising the arms or legs with ankle weights attached or resistance bands. Or even using your own bodyweight to exercise. Resistance training is about what you do and how you do it. Ninety percent of the battle is showing up mentally and physically.

Most people ask me questions about training, or book sessions to train with me, only after something has happened. They went to the doctor's office and he said they have to start working out because of this medical condition or that one. My question is: why did you have to let it get so far gone before you paid into yourself? I can tell you, NO amount of money will help you get the quality of life you deserve when health issues arise and take hold of your body. You may have money to address the problem, but not correct it, if your condition is terminal.

Get started *before* your health is an issue. Be proactive and preventative. Use focus and self-discipline to begin a fitness program early on and prevent yourself from ever having to combat an issue. Train right from the beginning.

It is my goal as a certified fitness trainer, sports nutrition specialist, martial art instructor, and martial artist, to use my 32 years of weight training experience with 30 years of martial arts training and teaching to compile a comprehensive book made for the average person and martial artist. This book is written and created for life transformation. For long-term growth and continued strength gains.

There are no shaky fundamentals, backward foundations, and shortcut principles here. Through my many years of resistance and martial arts training, I have learned that the only way to truly succeed in life, or in anything you do is through focus, mental visualization, hard work, discipline, self-control, and self-determination. I honestly believe that nothing printed in this text will be of benefit to you unless *you* make the choice to change. *And stick with it!* Believe me, if it were easy, everyone would have those million-dollar bodies you see on TV (without cosmetic surgery), and my life would have been a lot easier, with less WORK!

Unless you are new to resistance training, some of the information in this text is not earth-shattering or new resistance or weight training information. This is the tried and true information I've been using for over 30 years to teach clients and students where to turn when they hit a plateau. These are my personal resistance training and program documents that I've given to family, friends, students, and clients as reference materials. I can assure you this information has been life tested by me for the last 32 years and will continue to be used for my continued growth and development. It is my personal goal in creating this book that you don't repeat some of the same mistakes I've made in trying to get that perfect body (or should I say, other people's perception of the perfect body) without the hard work it takes to achieve it and keep it!

I've included sections on how and why you should resistance train as well as do other workouts to get you started. There are even motivations and quotes to help you stay on track and move forward. This book is designed to guide you through resistance training and start you well on the road to a healthy, active lifestyle that will keep you fit and strong. Something everyone needs. Keep moving. Keep achieving. Keep improving.

CHAPER ONE: GETTING STARTED

"Where Do I Really Begin?"

To reduce the risk of injury, there are some basic rules you need to follow. These rules apply to EVERYONE, whether you're getting back into a training program after a break or are getting started as a first-timer. (Sometimes we forget what got us there and go right for the gusto without taking our time!) Regardless of your age, you need to follow these rules.

Some basic rules of fitness:

1. Warm-up properly before you stretch. Warm-up before your strength or fitness training. This is your body's ramp up time, you don't want to get injured. Skipping your warm-up can lead to injury. Skipping your stretching after your workout slows down your recovery process.

Joint Rotations

- Beginning at your fingers and working down to your toes (being sure to include the neck) or working from your toes upward, rotate each joint to stimulate the flow of synovial fluid (joint lubricant).

- Rotate joint clockwise and counterclockwise until movement is fluid and free
- Fingers
- Wrists
- Elbows
- Shoulders
- Neck
- Hips
- Knees
- Ankles
- Toes

Aerobic warm-up

- 3-5 minutes of cardiovascular activity to raise your body temperature and to stimulate blood flow to your muscles
- Now that your body is properly warmed up with good flexibility, you're ready to stretch.

2. Stretch - for a list of suggested stretches, see Chapter 2: Do I Really Need to Stretch? The answer is 'Yes!' Follow the instructions outlined there.

3. Train your body parts by groups working larger muscles first (i.e. Chest) to the smaller ones (shoulders and triceps). Your quads, hamstrings, glutes, and pecs are huge muscles, you want to work all of them before your abs, deltoids, triceps, and biceps.

4. Try not to train the same body part two days in a row. (ex. Chest on Monday and Chest on Tuesday)

5. Don't max out every workout! (Your body needs time to heal, adapt, and recuperate.)

6. Try and rest for at least 45 - 60 seconds between sets. This will give you time to recharge for maximum lifts. You're recharging your

brain as well as your body. Focus your mind on your next set. Psych yourself up. If you are training for competition, take a 30-second rest so you can get used to recovering faster with less time! And again, put yourself in the right mind frame. You can do this!

7. Have a plan when you begin your routine. Use a workout schedule that breaks down each body part and training routine into sets. How many times you will do that exercise and reps - meaning how many times will you perform that movement, rest, then repeat it again.

8. Train within your range. In other words, an increase in logical, practical increments. Don't jump from 1-20 reps overnight. Or 10 to 40 lbs either. When training with a partner, don't try to train at their pace if you know you can't keep up. Take your time and find your limit to train smart and safe. Always concern yourself with injury prevention first.

9. Follow your work out with a final stretch. This enhances muscle flexibility and reduces muscle tension. You'll be less likely to be sore and, therefore, more likely to want to work out next time.

10. Use common sense.

These are *rules*. They are not flexible. By following them, you are giving yourself the best chance to prevent injury. There are other rules that could be added here but these are the most basic, most important ones to follow every day with every workout. Add your own rules as you see fit. Add your gym rules. Keep them in mind at all times, especially the last one, #10: Use common sense.

TERMINOLOGY

Now let's understand the basic terms used in this industry daily.
Fitness, *noun,* the condition of being physically fit and healthy.
The general components of fitness are:

1.) Agility - The ability to be quick and graceful;

2.) Cardiovascular Endurance - the ability to exercise without becoming overly tired because of the efficiency with which your heart, lungs, and blood vessels deliver oxygen to your body tissues.

3.) Cardiorespiratory Endurance - the level at which your heart, lungs, and muscles work together when you're exercising for a period of time.

4.) Balance - the ability to stay in control of body movement, with an even distribution of weight, to remain upright and steady

5) Coordination - The ability to move two or more body parts under control, smoothly and efficiently.

6) Explosive Strength - an individual's ability to exert a maximal amount of force in the shortest possible time.

7) Flexibility - the quality of bending easily without breaking, the ability to move through a full range of motion.

8) Speed Endurance - simply means how fast you perform something.

9) Strength Endurance - simply means how long you can stay strong while performing something.

10) Strength - the quality or state of being physically strong.

11) Body Mass Index (BMI) - how much fat do you have? See more on this below.

12) Range of Motion (ROM) - the full movement potential of a joint or body part.

13) Deconditioning - the reversal of previously conditioned behavior. In other words, the failure of your muscles to maintain the strength you brought them up to because you failed to keep them in condition.

14) Aerobics - vigorous exercises, such as swimming or walking, kickboxing, soccer, running - any exercise that gets your heart beating - designed to strengthen the heart and lungs.

15) Maximum Heart Rate (MHR) - the maximum amount of beats your heart will beat in one minute. It is used to calculate your target heart rate zone.

16) Exercise Benefit Zone (EBZ) - the phase in your body where your metabolism starts burning energy.

17) Rep or repetition - an exercise movement performed by lifting a weight from the start to the top of the movement and back down again.

18) Set - A series of single repetitions done in succession and then terminated.

19) Super Set - two sets for the same or different muscles without resting in between.

20) Tri-sets - three sets performed in a row with no rest.

21) Circuit training - one *giant set* performed with no rest at all until the prescribed number of sets is complete.

22) RM - Repetition Maximum - the most weights you can lift for a specified number of repetitions. I.E. 10RM = 10 repetition maximum. You can lift that weight 10 times before you fail. Your arms are shaking, you're straining. Maybe you have to hold your breath to continue.

BODY FAT

Fat is necessary to maintain life and reproductive functions. The amount of essential body fat differs between men and women and is typically around 2-5% in men, and 10-14% in women. The healthy range of body fat for men is typically defined as between 8-19%. While the healthy range of body fat for women is higher at 21-33%. The reason women store more fat than men is that at some point in their lives many women will need that fat to nurture a fetus, especially during the last two trimesters of pregnancy. These fat ranges change with age, especially after the '40s.

Body fat is, believe it or not, training fuel. It's what your body burns as you train. Professional and superior amateur athletes often have a body fat percentage much lower than the average person. For example, male marathon runners have been found to have an average body fat level of 8.5, but some have body fat as low as 3 percent. I can attest to this due to the fact that when I was competing in TaeKwon-Do tournaments I stayed between 6-7% body fat. Female marathon runners have an average body fat level of 8.5 but have been found to have body fat as low as 9.5 percent. When a woman's fat deposits get too low, she will cease to menstruate.

The Body Fat Calculator can be used to estimate your total body fat based on specific measurements. Here is the link: https://www.calculator.net/body-fat-calculator.html. Choose male or female. You enter your age, weight, height, neck, waist, and hip measurements then hit calculate. Your results can be calculated in the US, Metric, or Other units.

Use this chart:
https://www.nhlbi.nih.gov/health/educational/lose_wt/BMI/bmi_tbl.htm to quickly calculate your *Body Mass Index* (BMI) - a measure of body fat based on height and weight. This one is calculated on a quick chart according to your height and weight.

However, to accurately obtain your body fat amount, you must go to a dietitian to really give you your exact percentage. If you are using any other method, you'll be off by a few percentage points.

NOW HERE COMES THE TRAINING:

When you hear the term "PUMP" or "PUMPED" it means that a muscle is experiencing a massive flow of blood to it.

The "BURN" is lactic acid build up in the muscle. You will feel a tingling, burning sensation that tells you you have worked that muscle hard.

Over Training

When your body ceases to make progress, you have overtrained. The causes of overtraining are either too great a frequency, too great an intensity, or too great a duration of an exercise over a given period of time. To avoid this, set training times between 30 minutes to an hour maximum for each workout session. If you walk into a gym and are spending an hour and a half to two hours of training the same body parts, something in your routine needs to change to avoid overtraining.

Aerobics

Aerobics are vigorous exercises, such as swimming or walking, kickboxing, soccer, running - any exercise that gets your heart beating - designed to strengthen the heart and lungs.

Frequency, duration, and intensity. Frequency refers to how often you perform the aerobic activity. Duration refers to the time spent at each session. And intensity refers to the percentage of your maximum heart rate, or heart rate reserve, at which you work.

Little known fact: after reaching your maximum heart rate (MHR) for your exercise benefit zone (EBZ), the phase in your body where your metabolism starts burning energy, your body will stay in the fat-burning mode of up to 6 hours. Don't believe me? Ever have a great work out and take a shower, but you're still sweating for at least an hour or two afterward? That's your body killing it and remaining in the EBZ zone.

Injury

Should you suffer from an injury at any time, your first course of action should be to immediately stop your activity. Then use this formula R.I.C.E.: Rest, Ice, Compression, and Elevation. Rest your injury. Apply ice. Apply compression in the form of a bandage or wrap being sure not to cut off circulation. Then Elevate your injury. Some pains, such as muscle soreness, benefit instead of heat - like a hot tub or warm shower. But these are not generally injuries but are, rather, simply soreness. Injuries generally involve swelling and need ice.

After this initial treatment, if you do not see improvement within 24 hours, consult a physician. Take their advice. Do not return to your work out routine while you are suffering pain. Nothing good can come of it. In fact, that is the way to chronic pain, chronic injury. If you are a young person, you do not want this to become a life-long injury so please, follow your doctor's advice and wait out your healing period.

When you've received the go-ahead, begin slowly. You are re-training. Your muscles have lost some of their conditioning. Allow them to recover by easing into your work out. You do not want to compound your troubles by re-injuring yourself or injuring something new.

BE certain you are using the correct technique, especially warm-up, pre, and post-workout stretching. No pain, no gain is *not* a truism. No effort, no gain *is*. Now get back out there and put your all into it. *Wisely!*

Notes: Before you begin any exercise, you have to do some stretches to prepare your body for the next form of exercise. Don't overdo your exercises otherwise, they will leave you drained. Train within your range and have a training routine to follow each day.

CHAPTER TWO: DO I REALLY NEED TO STRETCH?

"What you didn't know about the Benefits of Flexibility and Training"

Flexibility is a joint's ability to move through a full range of motion. Flexibility training (stretching) helps loosen and relax muscle groups that might be overused during exercise or physical activity or as a result of bad posture. It's important to clearly understand the many benefits that result from a good flexibility program. Here's a list of a few things flexibility training can improve.

1. Physical Performance
2. Decreased Risk of Injury
3. Reduced Muscle Soreness
4. Improved Posture
5. Reduced Risk of Low Back Pain
6. Increased Blood and Nutrients to Tissues
7. Improved Muscle Coordination
8. Enhanced Enjoyment of Physical Activities

As you can see from this list, stretching has many benefits. If the only one it did was the last one, enhancing your enjoyment of physical activities, wouldn't you want to do it? You picked up this book because you're interested in resistance and combat training - very physical activities. You obviously want to enjoy them. Stretching before you start is going to enhance that enjoyment so you're going to *want* to do it.

But the benefits don't stop there. You just put in ten minutes of stretching. So now you've increased the blood flow to your tissues which means improved muscle coordination, thus, lowering your chance of injury. You've also improved your posture. And those two things combined give you a better chance at a perfect form when you lift, all contributing to a decreased risk of injury. Now, you're able to put in a full and satisfying workout with the lowest amount of post-workout muscle soreness. All because you took the time to put in some flexibility training pre-workout. Smart man! Smart woman! Smart person!

When you stretch, your muscles adjust then fix themselves and record the results of that action for future use. The muscle fibers themselves act like little computers, i.e. the term 'muscle memory', to register where you last extended. This is good to know because when you've made it there once on the extension, your body acts like a safeguard to get you to that point again. It's extending past this point, without the proper time for the body to record new gains, that an injury could occur.

To create greater memory markers, use added resistance to certain stretch movements, either assisted by a partner or by weight resistance. Push the body's range of motion (ROM) past perceived markers slowly. This will prevent injury in the event that the body has to move in that manner unexpectedly or past your normal ROM, meaning those extension markers or muscle memory records will prevent the body from injuring itself when those muscles must perform "cold" (without a proper warm-up), like in a self-defense situation. You still have to practice these stretch routines at least three times a week for such benefits to take effect, otherwise, you could pull or strain those muscles due to inflexibility or basic deconditioning. In other words, you must stretch and increase your stretch so that your muscles will permit you to perform unexpectedly should the need arise.

Before stretching:

Perform joint rotations as outlined in Chapter 1 followed by an aerobic warm-up as suggested there. Once your joints are loose and lubricated and blood is flowing through your muscles and your body temperature is elevated (now properly 'warmed up'), you are now ready to proceed to stretch.

STRETCHING TECHNIQUES:

Some experts feel that many stretching exercises should be avoided but I have mixed feeling about some things on this list like:

1. Head Rolls

This can be full or half. In a slow, smooth motion, roll your head beginning at one shoulder, dropping forward, proceeding to move towards the other shoulder. For a full roll, proceed to roll the ear over the shoulder around to the back continuing all the way around to the original shoulder. Repeat several times. Reverse the direction.

For a half roll, you will do a front half and a back half. Simply drop the ear to one shoulder slowly and smoothly rotate the head forward and across the body until the ear is at the other shoulder. Pause. Then rotate the head back across the body to the original shoulder. That is the front.

This time, drop the head towards the back of the body and roll from shoulder to shoulder. Be slow, methodical, and gentle. That is the back half.

2. Arm Circles

Hold your arms parallel to the ground, palms down. Rotate arms forward for a count of ten. Reverse direction for a count of ten.

Variations:

Increase the size of the circles. Perform medium circles. And then very large circles which are the full range of motion of your arms. Reverse direction on each.

Try the same circles this time turn palms up. Also, reverse direction and size on each.

3. Waist Circles

Firmly plant your feet shoulder-width apart. Place both hands on your hips and circle in a smooth and steady manageable circle. Lean forward and begin to circle your upper body around and do not twist. Simply rotate in a circle. Be smooth and steady. This does not need to be as fast, simply moderate and smooth. Proceed around several times. Then reverse direction.

4. Backbends

The backbend is an extreme stretch, not for the beginner. But anyone can stretch their back *towards* a backbend. To start working towards a backbend, first, stretch out your hands and your back. You will need flexible fingers to begin with. Straighten your arm fully in front of you raising your fingers towards the ceiling. Gently pull your fingers back with your other hand. When you've gotten a satisfactory stretch, switch hands. When both hands are warmed up and you've stretched your lower back with other exercises such as cat/cow, cobra, bridge, and bow poses, you're ready to proceed with a wall backbend.

Place your hands on the wall stretched straight out. Now take one step further back. That's how far you should stand away from the wall. Turn around. Bend backward to place your hands over your head and against the wall. Slowly walk your hands down the wall until you begin to feel compression on your lower back. *Go no further!* This is your maximum stretch. After this point, you face injury.

Variation:

Bridge:

Lay on a mat with your arms at your sides, knees bent, slightly apart. Press your hips up, keeping shoulders to the mat.

5. Prone Arch

Lay on your stomach then lift both arms and legs off the mat at the same time. Hold.

6. Straight Leg Sit Ups or Feet Held Down

Sitting on a mat, put your arms across your chest with your legs stretched straight in front of you. Lay back. Pull yourself to return to the sitting position while extending your arms towards your toes. When you become fatigued, stretch your arms overhead and use their momentum to help you sit up.

Variation:

Have a partner hold your feet down. Otherwise, the move is the same as above.

7. Leg Lifts

Here I'll cover four types of leg lifts. As we've previously discussed, doing the same routine every time you workout can get boring and is one of the causes of gym drop-out. So variation is key.

<u>Straight leg lifts</u>: Lay on your back on the mat. Lift your legs straight off the floor, bending at the waist, rising towards the ceiling until they are perpendicular to your torso. Slowly lower back down until your legs are just an inch off the ground. Repeat.

If you experience any back pain, a rolled-up towel can be placed under your lower back for comfort.

This particular variation can be further varied by doing it on a bench for an increased range of motion and improved abdominal strength.

<u>Variation 1</u>: Bend your legs as you lift. Same movement. This is the easiest variation. Towel and bench variations apply as above.

<u>Variation 2</u>: Place a medicine or exercise ball between your feet and, with legs straight, proceed as in the straight leg lift explained above. This also can be done on a bench. The added weight gives resistance and requires extra effort from your abdominals. Be sure to maintain a slow, steady, controlled rhythm in your repetitions.

A variation on this variation is to lift your torso up towards your legs in a V-shape and pass the ball from your feet to your hands then lay back down and crunch back up once again. Repeat.

<u>Variation 3: Hanging Leg Lifts</u>. Hang from a bar with a firm hand grip a little more than shoulder-width apart. Face forward keeping your head and neck relaxed. Lift your legs from your waist with as little body movement as possible controlling the slow, steady movement with your abdominal strength. Raise your legs until they are parallel to the ground. Pause. Lower slowly. Repeat.

A variation on this is to bend your legs to lift. Vary again by lifting legs to the right side and then the left.

Let me remind you here that each of these variations needs to be done in a slow, steady motion with control at all times.

<u>Variation 4: Side Lying Leg Lifts</u>. Once again, you are on a mat. This time on your side, your body stretched out and aligned, lower leg slightly bent. Prop your head up with your elbow to keep from straining your neck. Your free hand can be placed on your hip or on the floor in front of you for balance. Lift and lower your upper leg with a steady movement. Keep the hips aligned and do not allow the upper hip to roll forward.

While this is a great leg exercise, working both the adductors and abductors (inner and outer thigh muscles), it also works the butt.

Vary the intensity of this exercise by adding ankle weights.

8. Straight Leg Toe Touch

These can be done both standing and lying. I'm going to explain the standing ones first. Use your body weight for a gentle stretch down towards your toes. After you've started a gentle stretch, you can proceed to the more active lying stretch.

Standing Straight Leg Toe Touch:

Stand with your legs spread wide. Begin with a slight twist in your waist as you lean down toward your opposite foot. Start with a gentle stretch that pulls slightly. Let yourself feel the warmth of this stretch in the back of the leg you are leaning towards, up over your entire back, down your opposite arm, even in your neck. Inhale and exhale slowly. As you exhale, reach ever so slightly further. Reaching too far too soon is how you injure yourself. This is a gentle, warming stretch - not a torture rack.

Slowly raise back up and lower to the other side or sweep to the other side. Repeat the same slow stretching on the other side.

Variation: Feet can be together. Round down slowly collapsing the spine one vertebrae at a time until the upper body hangs from the waist with the weight of it pulling the spine and lengthening it to let the arms reach towards the toes. Let the weight of the body do the work of the stretch. Inhale and exhale slowly. With each exhale, allow the body to lower closer to the toes.

Lying Straight Leg Toe Touch:

Lift your legs into the air. Now stretch your arms towards your legs crunching up together. As you can tell, this is a much more active stretch than the standing toe touch. That's why it should be done *after* the standing one when your muscles are already warmed up. There is less chance of injury.

Variation 1: Spread your legs and lift one at a time to reach up to your hand. This also warms up your abdomen.

Variation 2: Hold both legs in the air spread apart. Reach towards one then the other alternately. This, too, warms up the abdominals.

9. Hurdle stretch (Do NOT attempt if you have knee problems)

Sit on a mat, one leg tucked behind your body on the floor, the other stretched before you, body bent forward over the front stretched leg. The hand on the side of the stretched leg will be supporting you on the ground. The other arm (the one on the side of the bent leg) is stretched out over the long leg towards the toe. You are in the position of a hurdler as he is mid-air jumping over the hurdle. Gently stretch your fingers towards your toe. Do not bounce but simply stretch forward. You will feel this stretch in your hip, groin, and abductors as well as the back. After a suitable stretch, say 30 seconds or longer, switch legs.

Variation 1: Seated Modified Hurdle. Sitting on the mat with legs stretched in front of you, tuck one foot up so the sole of the foot is pressed into the inner thigh of the opposite leg. Fold over your straight leg stretching your arms gently toward your toes. Remember to move slowly. Inhale. On the exhale, allow your muscles to relax towards the far toe. Inhale. Exhale and relax a further stretch, continuing for thirty or more seconds.

Variation 2: Standing Hurdle. This variation is vastly different from the others, not only because it is done standing, but also in the stretch it produces. Instead of stretching the back, it stretches primarily the inner thigh and the buttocks. Stand upright. Lift one leg to the front with the knee bent until it is parallel to the floor. Pivot it outwards to a 90 angle. Hold. Swivel back in. This provides stretch and balance.

10. Deep knee bends or squats.

For flexing and stretching, there should be NO motion past 90 when performing this exercise!!! More importantly, there should be no deep bends or bouncing of any sort!

Stand with feet hip-width apart, your toes pointed slightly

outward, hands laced behind your head. Pressing your heels into the floor and making sure they don't leave the ground, squat while bending slowly at the waist until your thighs are just past parallel to the floor. If you feel strain in your knees, reverse at parallel. Rise back up by squeezing the glutes and thrusting the hips forward. To avoid injury, do not bounce at the bottom of this move but reverse in a smooth motion to rise back up to a stand. This is a dynamic warm-up for glutes, quads, and calves increasing blood flow to these important muscles which help prevent injury when they come into use in important sports work like jumping, kicking, and running.

11. Calf Stretch

Seated Calf Stretch with a Resistance Band. Wrap the band around the ball of your outstretched foot as you sit on a mat. Bend the other knee up to rest on the bottom of its foot. Pull the band gently towards your face to stretch the calf and the foot. Naturally, you'll want to switch to the other leg to stretch both sides. No resistance band? Use a towel instead.

Heel Drop Stretch. Stand on a step with your heel hanging off with your toe on the step. Stretch heel down gently. Do not overstretch, especially when you are first beginning this move, as there are tendons attached to the heel that can rip. This is a gentle pressure and should just create the lightest tension.

Straight Leg Calf Stretch. Place hands flat against a wall stretched straight in front of you. Step your left leg back, bending the right knee. Slow lower the left heel to the ground behind you stretching the back of the calf. Hold at the point when you're feeling some tension. Do not overstress. These are delicate tendons.

12. Splits

Front Splits. This is easiest done in socks. Start in a low lunge. Place hands on either side of hips and point back toes resting the top of the foot on the ground. Glide the front foot forward while easing the hips towards the mat. Support hips on fingertips. Inhale. During the exhale, relax muscles towards the floor providing a gentle stretch downward. Inhale while holding the stretch. Exhale while allowing the muscles to gently relax towards the floor. Repeat as needed for a thorough stretch.

To release from this position, tilt hips towards the buttocks of the front leg and roll back leg forward in a semicircle.

Repeat the entire motion with the legs stretched in opposite directions.

Straddle (Chinese) Splits. When you have fully prepared your inner thigh muscles with butterfly stretches, lunges, and various other stretches, you are ready to attempt the straddle, middle, center, or Chinese splits - the many names for the same splits.

Again, as with front splits, this is easiest done in socks. Get down into a low squat with your hands on the mat in front of you. Slide your feet out parallel to the ground, keeping your toes pointed forwards. Keep your back straight and your hips in line with your legs. Do not allow your toes to turn upwards until you are in a full split position. You may not reach this position as it is very advanced. If you do not, simply hold the stretch while supporting yourself with your hands. Inhale. On your exhale, relax further into the stretch. Repeat several times. With practice, your stretch will improve.

Most of these exercises are part of many martial arts training programs or systems. When stretching, your thought process should be about moving at a gradual pace. Like everything else, you slowly work your way through stretching your muscles for maximum growth potential. Will you be masterful at stretching in such a short amount of time or even within a number of years? No. Not right off. But it is worth the effort! Improvements come gradually. You will see your progress. You will feel your progress.

POST WORKOUT STRETCHING

Just a few words on Post Workout Stretching. A lot of your work out has shortened your muscles. Stretching helps lengthen them back out to an elongated, relaxed position. They have also produced lactic acid and endorphins. As you stretch after your workout, you slow down the cooling process helping to release the lactic acids and endorphins thus alleviating any stiffness or soreness you might otherwise feel.

It's especially important after a burn out to bring blood flow back to muscles with a slow cool-down stretch. Your muscles need that oxygen. After all, you want to be able to continue using them even though you've just burned them out.

Your Post Workout Stretch helps reduce the risk of injury by improving your range of motion and easing tension from any over-worked muscles. So be sure to end every work out with a post-workout stretch. It's good for your whole body.

You can use these same stretches and many others to cool down with. See the example stretches in Chapter 10: How to Organize Your Resistance Training Routine for Beginners, Intermediate, and Advance Athletes for some post-workout stretching ideas.

As a professional instructor and trainer, I feel that after 30 years of martial arts training, many of these exercises have their benefits to the athlete - if performed properly! No exercise benefits anyone *unless it's done correctly!* I hope I've emphasized that enough by now.

NOTES: Stretches are very important as they help you to loosen and relax your muscles. If you have strained muscles, stretching will relieve the pain, reduce muscle soreness, and improve your physical performance during exercises.

A 10-minutes of stretching will increase blood circulation and make you feel better. Some of these stretches you can do include head rolls, arm circles, waist circles, straight leg sit-ups, etc.

CHAPTER THREE: THE AEROBIC VS. ANAEROBIC TRAINING EFFECT FOR CARDIOVASCULAR ENDURANCE

"To Breathe or Not to Breathe, understanding this now will affect your muscle performance"

Simply put, aerobic means with oxygen and anaerobic means without oxygen. Each energy system produces adenosine triphosphate (ATP), which is used by the muscles to contract. The aerobic system can utilize carbohydrates, proteins, or fat to supply an unlimited amount of ATP as long as oxygen is present. The aerobic system is used to power a steady state of exercise of continuous duration for longer than 3 to 4 minutes. Aerobic capacity is increased through interval training, continuous training (this must be intense enough to overload the aerobic system), and combat training.

The anaerobic system can only utilize carbohydrates for ATP production. This system does not use oxygen in the metabolization of its fuel source. The anaerobic system provides a short duration of exercise (45 to 70 seconds) and high power. The by-product of the metabolization of glucose (glycolysis) in this system is heat and lactic acid, the cause of muscle soreness immediately after exercise. Muscle soreness 24 to 48 hours after exercise is due to torn muscle fibers and connective tissue. Basic warm-up and cool-down stretching exercises can reduce this type of soreness. (See Chapter 2: Do I Really Need to Stretch?)

Anaerobic exercise is a type of exercise that breaks down glucose in the body without using oxygen. Anaerobic exercise is fueled by energy stored in your muscles through a process called glycolysis. Anaerobic exercise is an intense workout, while aerobic exercise is a long endurance workout. Anaerobic means with "no oxygen". All you need to understand is how the body uses energy. In anaerobic exercises, the body burns simple carbohydrates. In aerobic training, the body uses oxygen for energy. Note: your body will fall into both these phases for energy use while training, it just depends on what type of training you are doing.

Anaerobic activities consist of short exertion, high-intensity movement such as heavy weight training, mountain biking, jumping, sprinting, jumping rope, combat (martial and self-defense) training, sparring and grappling, and HIIT (High-Intensity Interval Training). In the anaerobic activity, your body requires immediate energy for maximum effort. It relies on stored energy sources for fuel, rather than oxygen. That's where the glucose breakdown comes in. Anaerobic activity is when you're working at about an 8 to 9 on a scale of one to 10 effort. You're working hard.

Whatever muscle group you choose to work anaerobically, you need to allow at least one day's rest for recovery. If you choose a full-body anaerobic workout, such as mountain biking, grappling, etc., allow a full day of recovery for your whole body.

Aerobic activities are cardiovascular activities that increase the heart rate such as swimming, jogging, hiking, biking, brisk walking, skiing, dancing. Your breathing and heart rate increase for a sustained period of time. This increase helps strengthen the heart, making it more efficient. As you can see by many of the exercises listed, anyone can participate in aerobic activity. And you can easily increase the level of your aerobic activity into anaerobic activity by increasing the intensity. It remains in an aerobic state as long as you're able to continue to take in oxygen. The easy way to calculate this is if you are able to carry on a conversation. You may have to gasp a bit, but you can still talk. When you can no longer keep up a conversation at all, you are in an anaerobic state. No oxygen.

Recommendations vary, but in short, anyone can benefit a great deal from a three days a week, 20 to 30-minute work out session no matter what age you are and when you start training! (See Conclusion for the American College of Sports Medicine guidelines on frequency of exercise to maintain cardiorespiratory and muscular fitness.)

Be sure to follow the chapter on stretching (Chapter 2: Do I Really Need to Stretch?) before any aerobic exercise - before exercise of any kind - to minimize muscle damage that can cause post-workout soreness that might discourage you from coming back for your next workout. Those 20 to 30 minutes, three days week workout sessions are just the minimum you need to keep your heart healthy. To improve muscle tone, to participate in active sports, to participate in MMA, combat training, or boxing, you're going to need a whole lot more. You *must* move into anaerobic conditioning.

As a beginner first entering a training program, start with aerobics, and build up your endurance. When you're ready to pack on the strength, that's when anaerobic comes in. Also, if you're trying to lose weight, anaerobic is crucial. HIIT (High-Intensity Interval Training) can help you meet these goals, as well as the resistance training thoroughly covered in the next chapters in this book.

The Benefits of Aerobic Exercise

- Improve your heart health
- Improves stamina and reduces fatigue
- Lower and control blood pressure
- Activate the immune system helping you fight colds and flu symptoms
- Boosts mood
- Has been attributed to longer life
- Improves your sex life (yeah!)

Because aerobics increases your heart rate, you should consult your doctor before starting an aerobics program, particularly if you've been inactive for a long time.

Benefits of Anaerobic

- endurance - when you do anaerobic training, your other workouts get easier
- Improved VO2 max (Maximum oxygen uptake)
- Improved weight loss
- strengthens bones
- burns fat
- builds muscle
- increases stamina for everyday activities like playing games or playing with your kids
- This one also improves mood

Consult with a fitness professional to be certain your anaerobic program is in harmony with your medical history. Be certain to perform all activities with the correct technique. Progress slowly and wisely and according to your own fitness needs, not someone else's. And please keep in mind all the rules put in place in Chapter 1: Getting Started.

HIIT (HIGH-INTENSITY INTERVAL TRAINING)

High-Intensity Interval Training is a combination of intense workout (at about a level 9 out of 10 in perceived exertion) followed by rest or low-intensity work. You're working balls-to-the-wall. Iron man style. This is your defining moment. But you've only got to do it for 30 to 90 seconds. You can do that. You got this, man!

And then you get to rest. Or at least slow down. And after that level of killer effort, anything seems like a rest.

The low-intensity rest periods allow the body to prepare for the high-intensity work, maximize calorie burning, and maximum muscle building. A good HIIT ratio is 1:2 for a beginner. Rest twice as long as you work at maximum intensity. If you choose to sprint for 30 seconds, rest for 60 seconds, then sprint again. And so on. When you're more experienced, switch to a 1:1 ratio. Power lift the most intense weights you can safely lift for 90 seconds, then rest for 90 seconds. Repeat. You're a monster! Do it again! Smash that weight out! Pump it! Pump it! 90 seconds! Rest! Whew! You did it. You killed it!

And the benefits will stay with you for hours. Your body is a calorie-burning mega-machine.

Your HIIT workout can last for 20 to 45 minutes. Three times a week is a good goal. You need at least one day's recovery between workouts for your body to rebuild. That doesn't mean you have to rest entirely. You can do aerobics if your workout was with weights, or weights if your HIIT workout was sprints or another kind of non-weight bearing workout.

HIIT workouts benefit you in that they continue calorie-burning post-workout due to increased metabolism. Because HIIT is a powerful workout, burning calories for long after you've finished your routine, be sure to eat a well-balanced and nutritious diet to keep up your strength for your next routine. This includes high protein and carbs.

HIIT WORKOUTS

Here are a couple of workout ideas for you to try:

Sprint

This HIIT can be done on the ground or on a treadmill. Do a three-minute jog to warm up. Now for the high-intensity part: balls-to-the-wall, hard as you can, superman style race for your life for 20 seconds. It's only 20 seconds. You can do it. Push. Push. Push.

Using the 1:2 ratio, you now rest for 40 seconds. Consult your trainer on this. Some may recommend a longer rest interval. If you're more advanced and doing a 1:1 ratio, only rest for 20 seconds before getting back to it.

Back to your sprint and your most intense level of effort. Go at it full tilt!

Repeat this pattern for 15 minutes of good solid workout - or more, depending on your trainer's instructions and your workout goals.

For a variation, do your sprints up a hill.

Tabata Protocol

With this HIIT exercise, you'll be using a bodyweight resistance move. You get to pick your favorite one. Let me suggest mountain climbers as an example. Although the walking gecko crawl is one of my personal favorites, it is difficult to do at high intensity while maintaining good form. So let's go with mountain climbers.

This is going to be difficult. That's the point. You're building unbelievable strength and endurance here. That takes work and sacrifice. The cool thing is - you only have to kill it for *four* minutes. You can do that, right? And it's not even four *straight* minutes. It's 20 seconds. Then a rest. You absolutely *can* do that. And when you're done, you can proudly say, 'Yes, I killed it!"

Mountain climbers, as hard and as fast as if you were being chased by a wild bear and your only escape is up the mountain - fast! 20 seconds. Kill it!

Rest for 10 seconds. You know what comes next: do it again. Keep up this pattern for 8 sets. You just beat the bear!

For a variation, do spiderman climbers on every other set. Remember, in this variation of the mountain climber, your knee comes to the outside of your arms and your foot can touch down or ride high (more challenging) before returning to start.

Substitute stationary bike, battle ropes, or sled for any of the intense part of the workout in the above examples. And a body resistance movement of your choice. But don't limit yourself to single move HIIT workouts. HIITs can also be multi-move. For example: Do as many pull-ups as possible in 30 seconds followed immediately by 60 jumping jacks then 20 burpees. Now rest.

Try mixing jumping rope in with your favorite body resistance moves like push-ups, planks, and resistance band squats. So you would Jump rope for 30 seconds then immediately do 10 push-ups, jump rope for 30 seconds, into 30 seconds of plank, jump rope for 30 seconds, and then 10 resistance band squats. Now rest.

You get the idea. Don't be static. Use your creative powers. Remember, gym dropout is prevented by an interesting workout. The more varied your program, the more likely you are to stick to it.

NOTES: Aerobic exercises utilize carbs, protein, and fat to provide you with the oxygen required to do the exercises. In aerobic exercises, the body uses oxygen for energy. While anaerobic exercises help break glucose in the body without using oxygen. Your body uses the energy stored in the muscles.

Both forms of exercise offer different benefits to your body. For example, Aerobic exercises improve your heart health, control blood pressure and increase stamina. Anaerobic exercises aid in weight loss and strengthen your bones.

CHAPTER FOUR: THE FACTS ABOUT RESISTANCE TRAINING FOR WOMEN

"Resistance Training = Strength Training = Body Shaping"

For years, doctors have advised women to engage in aerobic and weight-bearing exercises to increase their bone mass. Such training helps to delay the onset of symptoms and, in some cases, prevent osteoporosis. Bone loss begins as early as age 35 and can massively increase following menopause. But interestingly, recent studies have shown that resistance training is also effective at increasing bone density, and, in fact, maybe more effective than aerobic training. Muscle strength and balance were also improved in resistance-trained women.

An Australian study of postmenopausal women divided them into three groups. One group engaged in strength training, one in fitness, and one in no exercise at all. All were given calcium supplements. Though both the strength and fitness groups experienced increases in their bone mineral density, the strength training group had a greater increase in bone density at the vulnerable hip joint.

One study of postmenopausal women participating in a weight training program for a year showed an increase in density of the bones in the spine and hips, the areas most affected by osteoporosis. One of the most critical concerns with osteoporosis is fractures caused by falling. Weight training (resistance training) increases balance and coordination thus preventing such falls.

The mortality rate of a woman who has had a hip fracture increases five to eight times above that of her compatriots. Therefore, the prevention of falls in the first place is crucial. You can help yourself by improving your coordination with resistance and other training and prevent the chance of fracture with resistance training that increases your bone density.

As we age, we lose muscle mass, as much as 55% by the time we're 70 years old. That's why old people often feel so weak and tired. Resistance training helps keep up muscle mass to prevent that. Therefore, it has long-term health benefits. Start young and continue for a lifetime.

The back - the entire spine - and hips are key areas of concern for osteoporosis prevention but osteoporosis is a bone disease and affects all bones so weight lifting should be done throughout the entire body to prevent and reduce it. There are other risk factors involved so, as with other medical concerns, consult your doctor for more information and further preventative measures.

Here are some reasons, in addition to building strong muscles why women should strength train:

- Building toned, beautiful muscles
- Lower risk of heart attack or stroke (2018 study by Iowa State University showed that just an hour a week can lower risk by 40 to 70 percent)
- Improve insulin sensitivity (research shows that women who lift just twice a week are less likely to develop Type 2 diabetes)
- Reduce inflammation (Mayo Clinic study)
- Reduce anxiety and depression (Duke University study showed that clinically depressed patients were able to manage symptoms *without* medication when undergoing weight lifting four times a week for four months)
- Improves focus (Archives of Internal Medicine participants who weight trained did better on cognitive tests than those who focused on balance and toning)

- Improves chance of survival (2014, University of California Los Angeles study showed that more muscle mass lowers the chance of premature death. Huh. Who knew? (wink, wink)

The big question most women have concerning resistance training is 'Will I bulk up?' The simple answer is no. You have estrogen. That wonderful feminine hormone that prevents you from looking like a man - *ever*. You will see firm, feminine toning. Not masculine muscles. You will improve your strength and endurance as men do.

Like a man, you can overwork a muscle. You can make it out of proportion to other parts of your body. But that takes a lot of effort. Follow the wise advice I give you in this chapter and elsewhere in this book and you will simply see toned, feminine curves that will keep you fit, healthy, and strong. Few women can work any of their muscles into anything resembling something masculine. Don't worry.

We've all seen Aunt Sally waving across the yard and that flabby flap of skin under her arm jiggling away like some loose dog's jowl. Yuck! Had Aunt Sally been doing a little resistance training - anything from a few wall push-ups every day to milk jug curls to full-on deadlift to fatigue - she wouldn't be sporting those mud flaps. And we wouldn't be witnessing those eyesores.

That's what weight training can prevent you.

Strength training helps you preserve lean muscle mass which diminishes with age. It's the lean muscle mass that burns calories, helping keep your weight in check. Of course, all those strong muscles support your bones and improve your balance, thus preventing injury. However, it's up to you to use good training techniques and proper form to make sure the lifting itself doesn't injury you. Always remember to increase weights gradually. And if an added weight feels too heavy, don't hesitate to remove it. Don't let your ego stand in your way. Better to step back down and lift a lower weight to fatigue than to injure yourself and be down for the count until you recover.

GETTING STARTED IN RESISTANCE TRAINING

Body Weight

Using your own body weight for resistance is an excellent, inexpensive, readily available way to begin. Your body weight is available any time you are. And it's free. What could be better?

Here are a couple examples of some bodyweight resistance exercises:

Plank: Anyone can do a plank. You may not be able to sustain it for long the first time you attempt it but you will be able to build your endurance. It engages lots of muscles and it powers up your core. This is like a push-up except that you are on your elbows rather than your hands.

- Balance on your elbows and your toes
- Tuck your chin.
- Push your shoulder blades forward
- Tilt your pelvis in
- Extend your legs

You are now in the plank position. Hold. Engage your core. Breathe. Try to hold this position for 20 seconds.

Mountain Climbers: Lift into a push-up position. Bring one foot forward between arms then switch with the other foot. These can be done in rapid succession for an anaerobic workout. They can be done at maximum effort for part of a HIIT (High-Intensity Interval Training) work out.

Spiderman Mountain Climbers: This is the same move except that your leg comes to the outside of your hands. In one variation, your foot touches the ground. For a more challenging version, it remains in the air before returning to its original position. Like the Mountain Climbers, these can be done in rapid succession for aerobic work out or at maximum effort for part of a HIIT (High-Intensity Interval Training) work out.

Donkey Kick: On your hands and knees, lift one leg, bent, behind you until your thigh is parallel with the ground. Clench your buttocks hard. Return to the ground, gently touching down the knee. Repeat. Be sure to work the other leg an equal number of times.

Since you're already on your knees, convert to a *single-leg kickback* where your leg is stretched straight back behind you. Lift that leg up until it is even with your butt. Lower slowly to the top of the foot. Repeat. Switch to the other leg. This works your buttocks and thigh together. Make certain that this is a firm and controlled movement.

Now move that to a *standing-leg kickback*. The same movement only standing. Move to a side-leg kickback by kicking your leg in a controlled motion to the side. You can also move your leg across the front of your body. After numerous repetitions, work the other leg in whichever move you are performing.

Curtsy Lunge with Side Kick: Start with your feet hip-width apart. Step your right leg diagonally behind your left leg bending into a lunge, then push up sweeping your back leg out to a low kick - higher if you're looking for a more aerobic workout. Switch legs. Then repeat the sequence.

Rubber Tubing/Resistance Bands

Resistance Bands come in different strengths. Find quality ones of a strength that's appropriate for you.

Step on the middle of the bands to do bicep curls, side lateral raises, lunges, shoulder presses, and front raises.

Bicep Curls: Stand in the middle of the band, feet together with a tall straight body. Grip bands with palms facing outwards. Curl slowly up towards biceps with the elbows tucked in and slightly forward of the body. Return to start in a controlled motion. Repeat.

Side Lateral Raises: Stand in the middle of the band with feet together. Your hands will be holding the resistance bands at the sides of your body with palms facing your legs. Slowly lift out and away to shoulder height as though you have wings. Slowly lower to start. Repeat.

Resistance Band Lunges: You are in a basic lunge position. The band is under your front leg and held in both hands. You dip down to the bended knee (the back leg) easing tension on the band and then rise up using the band's resistance. Repeat.

Shoulder Press with Resistance Band: For this move, your feet can be together or hip-width apart. I prefer hip-width. Arms are extended from shoulders and bent upwards gripping bands. Bands should be taut. Press upwards to extend arms fully above the head. Return in a controlled manner to start position. Repeat.

Front Raises: Stand on band with feet about a foot apart, knees slightly bent. Grip band in each hand firmly with hands next to legs hanging in a natural position. You will lift arms straight out and away from the body as you pull the band up to shoulder height. Slowly lower back down to start. Then repeat.

String over the head to a door or other attachment to perform tricep extensions, standing row, and chest press.

Remember the kickbacks from body resistance? In that position, put the band under one hand, hook the foot on that same side into the handle of the resistance band and kick back with that foot for a glute extension. You get a great butt workout with the added resistance of the band.

Free Weights

So many beautiful exercises to do with free weights. You can get a whole body workout in just three moves with free weights by doing the bench press, squats, and the deadlift. Three powerful moves with the powerful potential to build beautiful muscle. Done wrong, they can cause painful injury. So be certain you are using the excellent form and the right weight for your body and condition. See Chapter 10: How to Organize Your Resistance Training Routine for Beginners, Intermediate, and Advance Athletes for details on the proper form for each of these three essential moves.

Bench Press

Working this muscle gives your cleavage the same beautiful lift and separation of a Victoria's Secret push-up bra without the underwire. It will keep your breasts higher longer than your girlfriend's neglected pecs. So bench press away!

In case, you didn't know it yet, you will notice on your very first lift that the bench press targets your triceps as well as your deltoids. The deltoids are that round cap over your shoulder that keeps your bra straps in place. Remember what I said at the beginning of this chapter: the feminine hormone estrogen keeps you from getting big bulky shoulders like a guy. No worries. You will simply get some nice definition and tone that is still entirely feminine.

Squat

While we'll be working other muscles, our primary focus here is the gluteus maximus. That's right - your butt. Want a beautiful backside? Powerful kicker? You need this move. Born with a pitiful sitter? No worries. Learn to squat like a pro and you'll be filling out your Levi's like J Lo before you know it.

Again, this is a muscle that gets an overlapping workout because the deadlift works this one too. However, in the squat, we're working the lower and inner parts of this muscle primarily. While in the deadlift, we're working the upper part and into the erector spine (lower back). As with all three of these moves, form is *everything*. The potential for injury is in every single move. So is the potential for powerful success. Beautiful booty is just a squat away.

You've worked your abs with the bench press. Let's work on them again. Cause you can never, ever work your abs too much.

Deadlift

Its nickname is "the king of weightlifting". Why? Because it works out so many muscles all by itself that it's pretty much a full-body workout. It's recovering your abs and glutes, of course, and it's getting to your obliques - the side abdominals. Then it's giving a powerful workout to all those muscles the other two didn't touch including your neck - seriously! It's working the all-important back muscles which must be strong for all the everyday movements you do. It works those huge muscles in your thighs, both front and back and inner (quadriceps, hamstrings, adductors). Then right down to your calves (gastrocnemius and soleus), both the larger and smaller muscles, so you'll have powerful muscles for quick starts and stops when you need them - this is especially important in sports such as martial arts, basketball, soccer, etc. where quick bursts of sudden energy are essential and especially quick lower leg movement.

Three movements with free weights and you've just covered almost every muscle in your body. Wow!

Weight Machines

The advantage to using a weight machine is that the movement is controlled for you. Therefore, there is much less chance of injury as it is much more difficult to perform the movement incorrectly. Every gym has a different selection of weight machines and they cover every different body part. Most gyms will provide you with an introduction to the machines when you first join and adjust you to the proper measurements for your body. Their initial weight assessments may not be entirely accurate so feel free to make further adjustments on your own.

Here are a few good ones to try:

- Leg Extensions - start with 10 to 15 repetitions
- Leg Curl - also 10 to 15 repetitions. We will use this number of repetitions throughout.
- Chest Press
- Lat Pulldown
- Mid Row
- Shoulder Press

You don't have to go to the gym to do a resistance workout but your body needs it for healthy bones and good muscle tone. All that strength keeps you coordinated and graceful as well as looking good.

You can do it aerobically and anaerobically. Because you can use your own body as your resistance, you can do it anywhere anytime for free, making resistance training one of the best forms of exercise you can do. Make it a regular part of your healthy lifestyle.

Notes: Women can engage in resistance training exercises to increase their bone mass and strength. As you age, you can lose muscle mass and incorporating some strength training exercises in your daily routine provides you with a lot of health benefits.

It also helps prevent osteoporosis in women, reduce inflammation, lower risk of heart attack, and improve insulin sensitivity. There are different types of exercises you can including resistance band lunges, bench press, squats, and deadlift.

CHAPTER FIVE: THE FACTS ABOUT RESISTANCE TRAINING FOR MEN

"Dedication = Resistance Training = Strength Training = Flat Stomach"

Resistance training offers several cardiovascular benefits. It can improve odds associated with heart disease risk factors. It is helpful in cardiac rehabilitation after a heart attack, and it can help prevent non-heart failure. A Canadian cardiac rehabilitation study looked at the effects of resistance training among men recovering from heart attacks.

All 57 of the participants underwent aerobic exercise rehabilitation, and all had resistance training at low, medium, or high intensity. Maximum strength increased in the low-intensity resistance group by 10%, 12% in the medium group, and 14% in the high-intensity group. Of note, 30 of the men had heart complications during the aerobic exercise (abnormal rhythms, chest pain, blood pressure rises or drops), but only one had cardiac problems during resistance training, demonstrating that not only was it beneficial, but perhaps safer.

Often thought of as a disease affecting women, osteoporosis affects men as well, especially those with unhealthy habits like consuming too much alcohol, smoking, getting too little vitamin D or calcium or exercise, and there is one other high-risk factor - race. If you're a white man, your risk of osteoporosis is increased.

If you read the chapter on women and resistance training, you know that resistance training, also known as weight training, is highly beneficial in the prevention of osteoporosis as it strengthens bones as well as increasing balance thus preventing falls which create fractures in affected bones - less of a problem in men than women.

What else does "resistance" train? Here are several quick reasons: it boosts metabolism, regulates insulin which helps with diabetes, improves posture, improves sleep, elevates mood, increases energy levels, lowers inflammation. All great reasons. But for you guys, here are the two most excellent reasons. It increases endurance and, best of all, it improves strength.

Power. That's what it's all about. That's what resistance training gives you. More and more strength. More power in everything you do. Whether it's playing with the kids or sex, you'll have more stamina, more strength, more coordination.

How do you get it? Below are some excellent examples of the various types of resistance training available from free and always available bodyweight resistance to costly weight machines provided in gyms. Try them all. Use a combination. Be sure to keep track of your program and increase carefully and consistently.

GETTING STARTED IN RESISTANCE TRAINING

Body Weight

Using your own body weight for resistance is an excellent, inexpensive, readily available way to begin. Your body weight is available any time you are. And again it's free. What could be better?

Here are a couple examples of some bodyweight resistance exercises:

Plank: As I said, anyone can do a plank. You may not be able to sustain it for long the first time you attempt it but you will be able to build your endurance. It engages lots of muscles and it powers up your core. This is like a push-up except that you are on your elbows rather than your hands.

- Balance on your elbows and your toes
- Tuck your chin.
- Push your shoulder blades forward
- Tilt your pelvis in
- Extend your legs
- You are now in the plank position.
- For men, there is an additional, vital step: hollow your upper body by rounding your back
- Breathe.

The hollow body position offers many benefits over the neutral one in that it activates the serratus anterior muscles. This helps you with a winged scapula and gives you greater push strength, especially helpful in martial arts for moves like a close-quarter strike or the famous one-inch punch. It's one of the most important muscles of the shoulder complex because it helps move the arms multi-dimensionally. It helps with every over-head move known to man (push-ups, bench press, etc.).

Push-up: What an amazing exercise! There are so many variations of this exercise that it can be done by the earliest beginner with very little fitness level to the most advanced trainee. The more upright you are in performing this exercise, the less your exertion. The closer to horizontal you become, the harder your effort. Also, the closer together your hands are the more difficult the exercise becomes.

- Balance your hands and toes with hands shoulder-width apart
- Hands should be spread comfortably
- Lower in a slow controlled manner until inches from the ground
- Push back to starting position

For variation, try an incline. Put your hands on a raised bench. Or for the beginner, a wall. Step back a few paces, place your hands on the wall and push away. The closer towards horizontal you go, the harder it will be.

Another variation is a bent knee position. In this position, be sure to tuck your pelvis in so that your back does not arch which can lead to a lower back injury.

To focus the push up on the chest, do a wide push up with hands spread further apart. This is especially effective if done on rings where arms are spread wide at the bottom and pulled together at the top of the movement thus engaging chest muscles in an optimal way.

To focus on the triceps, place hands close together beneath the chest during the push-up. The sphinx variation engages the triceps even more. For this variation, extend the closely placed hands forward slightly beyond your head then lower the elbows to the ground rather than the chest for the movement.

Target your shoulders by doing the pseudo planche push-up. From the standard push-up position, lean forward before lowering to the ground. The more you lean forward, the harder the movement gets. If you are really advanced, you can do the full planche push-up with your feet off the ground.

Another way to target the shoulders is the pike push-up which is a nearly vertical movement. In this instance, your butt is in the air and you are in a V position. For a really fun variation, place your feet up a wall and run them down it to lower your head to the ground, run them back up it as you push yourself back up to the extended position.

And, of course, there is the ever-popular clapping push-up. When you can do twenty regular push-ups competently, you're ready to proceed towards this one. The next step is to do an explosive push-up in which you lift off the ground. Don't attempt to clap yet. Simply lift off the ground. When you're successful with this for your twenty reps, go to the next step.

Conquering clapping push-ups:

- Master 20 standard push-ups
- Master 20 push-ups with an explosive lift - just lift hands off the ground with each one.
- Add clap
- Advanced: Clap in front and behind back in one move.

The Gecko Crawl: This is another variation of the push up which engages core strength, coordination, strength, and mobility. And it looks way cool. Kinda like spidey crawling across the floor. Get into your push-up position. Bringing opposite hand and foot forward - left foot, right hand - lower yourself as close to the ground as possible. Lift while moving forward and switching hand and foot a la spiderman. Then lower. Try to make this a smooth transition from side to side while lowering and raising from the push-up position. Try going backward. This takes some coordination and strength. It's a great HIIT move too.

My coverage of push-ups wouldn't be complete if I didn't mention archer push-ups. These are leverage push-ups in which you lean to the side over one arm while the other arm is extended. The further the lean, the harder it becomes. To make it even more difficult, remove the extended arm altogether, making this a one-armed push-up.

The final push-up variation, posterior chain push-up, is also called the back bridge push-up or backbend. It is an advanced move because of the flexibility required. For this move, lie on your back with your hands palm down on either side of your head, feet flat on the ground. Lift your pelvis towards the sky, arching your back, belly and shoulders up, allowing your head to tilt down relaxed towards the ground. Lower gently back down.

Rubber Tubing/Resistance Bands

Resistance Bands come in different strengths. Find quality ones of a strength that's appropriate for you.

Squats

Step over the middle of the bands to do overhead *squats* with your feet shoulder-width apart. The band is around your whole body braced in your arms above your head as you squat which promotes good form. Be sure your arms do not creep out in front of you but stay over your head for the entire movement. Keep your back straight. Toes turned out. Hinge at the hips. Squat till thighs are parallel to the ground. Use your glutes to pull you back up to a stand.

Bent-Over Row

Once again, stand in the middle of the band with your feet shoulder-width apart. Grab the band close to your ankles for good resistance. Bend at waist with back flat to slightly arched. Chin up. Squeeze shoulders back and together using your back for the action. Release in a controlled manner. Repeat.

Chest Press

Use the same wide leg stance in the middle of the band with a wide hand grip. Focus your movement on your elbows. Squeeze and lift to chest height and lower back down. Repeat.

Overhead Press

For your arms, use the wide leg stance and both hands shoulder-width apart inside the band. Press from shoulders up to full extension above head. Return to shoulders and repeat. This works the front and side of the deltoids. The next exercise will work the back of the deltoid.

Mock Rear Fly

Hands shoulder-width apart straight out in front of you with the band taut between them. Stretch arms out to the sides working the back of the deltoids. Return to start and repeat.

Free Weights

So many beautiful exercises to do with free weights. I'm a big fan of three key moves that give you a full body workout all by themselves: bench press, squats, and the deadlift. Three powerful moves with the powerful potential to build beautiful muscle. Done wrong, they can cause painful injury. So be certain you are using excellent form and the right weight for your body and condition. For proper form on these three moves, see Chapter 10: How to Organize Your Resistance Training Routine for Beginners, Intermediate and Advance Athletes.

Bench Press

First up: Bench press. This key move is what really gives strength to the upper body. It's the glamour move for the chest. Now, I know, you're working out for health, improved stamina, or any of a number of other reasons. But somewhere in the back of your animal brain is a little itch you can't deny and it's saying, 'I wanna look good.' The bench press is that guy's friend 'cause its primary target is the pec major - the macho muscle of the male physique.

The bench press also works those sweet little muscles *beneath* the pecs which curve around the ribs. They lead down to the abs which the bench press also works, muscles which our other two moves overlap because you can never, ever work your abs too often.

In case, you didn't know it yet, you will notice on your very first lift that the bench press targets your triceps as well as your deltoids. The deltoids are that round cap over your shoulder, guys, that make you look broad-shouldered and manly.

Squat

While we'll be working the other muscles, our primary focus here is the gluteus maximus. That's right - your butt. Want a beautiful back-side? Powerful kicker? You need this move. Born with a pitiful sitter? No worries. Learn to squat like a pro and you'll be filling out your Levis like David Beckham before you know it.

Again, this is a muscle that gets an overlapping workout because the deadlift works this one too. However, in the squat, we're working the lower and inner parts of this muscle primarily while in the deadlift we're working the upper part and into the erector spinae (lower back). As with all three of these moves, the form is *everything*. The potential for injury is in every single move. So is the potential for powerful success. Beautiful booty is just a squat away.

You've worked your abs with the bench press. Let's work on them again. Cause you can never, ever work your abs too much.

Deadlift

"The king". As I said earlier because it works out so many muscles all by itself that it's pretty much a full-body workout. It's re-working your abs and glutes, of course, and it's getting to your obliques - the side abdominals. Then it's giving a powerful workout to all those muscles the other two didn't touch including your neck - seriously! It's working the all-important back muscles which must be strong for all the everyday movements you do. It works those huge muscles in your thighs, both front and back and inner (quadriceps, hamstrings, adductors). Then right down to your calves (gastrocnemius and soleus), both the larger and smaller muscles, so you'll have powerful muscles for quick starts and stops when you need to - this is especially important in sports such as martial arts, basketball, soccer, etc. where quick bursts of sudden energy are essential and especially quick lower leg movement.

Three moves with free weights and you've just covered almost every muscle in your body. Wow! If it sounds like I am repeating myself ... I am. I have a feeling some men will skip over chapter four because they think it is for women only.

Weight Machines

The advantage of using a weight machine is that the movement is controlled for you. Therefore, there is much less chance of injury as it is much more difficult to perform the movement incorrectly. Every gym has a different selection of weight machines and they cover every different body part. Most gyms will provide you with an introduction to the machines when you first join and adjust you to the proper measurements for your body. Their initial weight assessments may not be entirely accurate, however, so feel free to make further adjustments on your own.

Here are a few good ones to try:

- Horizontal seated leg press
- Overhead press
- Cable bicep bar (good choice for burn out)
- Cable tricep bar (good choice for burn out)
- Rowing Machine (excellent for HIIT)

These are just a few machines to try. Remember to start with your largest muscles and work to the smaller muscles.

As you can see, you have lots of choices when it comes to resistance training. Try them all. Choose what works best for you. To avoid gym drop-out, vary your workout. Keep track of your progress. Stay motivated.

Notes: Resistance training offers a lot of cardiovascular benefits and can improve conditions associated with heart diseases. Men with unhealthy eating habits, smoking, and consuming too much alcohol are at high risk of suffering from osteoporosis.

Doing resistance training not only improves their health condition, it can also strengthen their bones and increase balance. Weight lighting in men can increase their endurance, coordination and help them have more stamina.

A combination of various body weights, resistance bands, and other free weight exercises will put you not only in great shape but also make you feel healthy.

CHAPTER SIX: THE FACTS ABOUT RESISTANCE TRAINING FOR PRE-TEEN/TEEN/ADULTS

"Consistency = Resistance Training = Strength Training = Weight Gains"

Just like any form of exercise, the main goal in dealing with children or young adults is to challenge their minds and abilities. Far too often in this "New World" of Social Media, Youtube, high tech cellular video games, and PC-based past times, we are using these instruments as mindless and motionless past time activities for our young people. From many conversations with parents and my students, video games or PC activities are the new forms of babysitting or childcare. Let's face it, it's easier to put a child in front of a video game or PC instead of taking the time to engage their mind or body after a long day's work. Childhood obesity is a proven and growing problem among our youth! Finding fun ways to get the youth to exercise is the goal!

But is strength training right for my child?

Even the Mayo Clinic endorses strength training for young people. As does the American Academy of Pediatrics. They suggest it is helpful for kids as young as seven. Why? What are the benefits? Well, for the most part, they're the same as for an adult: strong bones, healthy blood pressure levels, maintaining cholesterol levels, maintaining weight. Resistance training can counter the effects of a sedentary lifestyle which so many young people have today. But for those youths getting out there and participating in sports, resistance training helps strengthen their muscles to improve performance and prevent injury in their chosen activity.

As with anyone participating in resistance training, it helps with self-esteem and confidence.

Sixty minutes a day of physical activity is the minimum recommended by the Department of Health and Human Services. Resistance training is an excellent choice for three-times a week strengthening of bones and muscles.

Resistance training will not turn the obese child into a muscle machine. But a combination of diet and exercise will help the child lose fat and resistance training can be an excellent part of that exercise program that will strengthen bones and muscles contributing to improved self-esteem and self-confidence which will encourage the young person's continued participation in physical activities.

Weight training is about building muscles and strength as opposed to weightlifting and powerlifting which are about the maximum amount of weight being lifted. Bodybuilding is about building a specific, aesthetically perfect muscular physique. Young people should stay away from the intense training necessary for these competitive sports until their bodies have fully matured, which does not happen until they are well into their twenties. Muscle tone, as opposed to bulk, happens with lighter weights and higher repetitions. Parents and trainers should look out for any student trying to achieve a bulked-up 'superhero' body. This can be a sign of body dysmorphic syndrome or lead to the possible use of steroids.

A big fear of resistance training in young people is damage to the joints or growth plates. But according to the National Strength and Conditioning association "most injuries to young lifters are the result of poor training protocols, excessive loading, poorly designed equipment or lack of adult supervision, not fragile anatomy."

David Sandler, MS, CSCS, owner of StrengthPro, Inc., and consultant on National Geographic Channel's Super Strength, says 'it's free weights that will ultimately produce the best technique and posture and, consequently, muscle gains.' So try the free weights. But most professionals recommend starting with bodyweight resistance to build strength and coordination first remembering to perform good technique no matter what resistance method is used.

Here are four types of resistance training and several exercises in each type to get you started:

Body Weight Resistance

Always a good choice for everyone because it is impossible to lift too much since the maximum you can lift is your own body weight. Form, however, as always, is important. And your body is always available for a workout anytime, any place. Very convenient.

Many school gym programs traditionally included bodyweight resistance activities as part of their warm-up portion of the class including burpees, lunges, arm circles, bicycles, and crunches. Even jumping jacks.

The bodyweight resistance moves listed here are specifically geared towards young people in the aspect of their fun quotient. However, body resistance moves listed in the other chapters, Chapter Four: The Facts About Resistance Training for Women and Chapter Five: The Facts About Resistance Training for Men, are just as applicable to everyone. Please explore them and use them in your exercise routine. I cannot emphasize enough the value of bodyweight resistance. It is available to you *at all times*. And *it's free!*

Dead Bug

How do dead bugs look? Turned up on their backsides with arms and legs in the air, of course. And that's how you need to be to start this move. Arms straight in the air, knees bent. Now lower one arm down to the ground beside your ear as you exhale like a bug giving out its last breath while at the same time stretching out the opposite leg. Inhale and bring both limbs back to the starting position. Repeat on the other side as you exhale (dying once again).

Spiderman Push Up

In this push-up, as you lower yourself to the floor, bring one knee up to try to touch it to your elbow. Then return it to the position before attempting the same on the other side. Go spidey!

Windshield Wipers

Lie on your back spreading your arms out from your shoulders to keep your body stable. Lift your legs straight into the air perpendicular to the mat. Keep your core tight as you move your legs side to side in imitation of windshield wipers. Some very flexible young people with good core strength will be able to lower their legs all the way to the mat on either side. Lower only as far as you can do so with good control.

Crab Walk

Sit on the mat with legs bent. Press up with hands and feet to lift your butt off the ground. Now scurry around like a little crab forwards, then backward. What fun! And good exercise too!

Inchworm

We are having so much fun! Let's continue it with the inchworm. Stand tall with your feet just about hip-width apart. Bend over to touch the ground and start walking your hands out. Keep your core (that's your belly) tight and firm. Keep walking until you're as close to the ground as you can get. Then start inching your toes towards your hands. Keep going until your feet meet your hands. You're an inchworm now!

Frog Stand

Squat down with your hands in front of your feet. Press your knees against your slightly bent elbows. Lift up onto your toes then bend slightly forward until you can lift your toes all the way off the ground to balance on your hands. This is easy to master when you are young.

Once you've got it, try extending your legs straight out behind you. This is called a planche.

Rubber Tubing/Resistance Bands

Resistance bands are fun. It's like playing with a giant rubber band. Even adults love that kind of fun. While the resistance band exercises listed here are specifically geared towards young people, anyone can do them, as well as young people performing the resistance band exercises listed in Chapter Four: The Facts About Resistance Training for Women and Chapter Five: The Facts About Resistance Training for Men of this book.

Row the Boat (Deadlift)

Step on the resistance band in a wide-leg stance, bend towards your feet, grasp the band in both hands so that it is taut between feet and hands. With a back level, 'row' to a standing position, pulling the band to your crotch.

Bow and Arrow

Hold the band with one hand extended to the far side of the head and the other hand fairly close as though you were about to notch an arrow in a bow. Pull back on the band as though you were preparing to launch that arrow. Hold. Slowly release back to starting position. Caution: *Do not release the band. Keep it in your control at all times.*

Flamingo Hops

Step on the band with one foot. Hold taut in both hands. Keeping the band taut under your foot, hop, hop, hop

Frog Jumps

Very similar to the Flamingo Hops, but with both feet in the band and arms bent to the sides of the chest. Hop, hop, hop, little froggies.

Fearless Warrior (Chest Flies)

Hold the band at chest level with hands fairly close together. Spread and stretch to a straightened (elbows slightly bent), wide-armed position. Controlling the motion, return to start. Feel free to groan 'Aaarrrgh', like a Fearless Warrior. (Or whatever sound makes you feel powerful.)

Free Weights

A good starting weight is one that you can easily lift ten times with the last two repetitions becoming more and more difficult. When those two are also easy, increase your weight. If you struggle to get to ten, you need to lower down your weight to something lighter. All the exercises listed in this section use dumbbells. These exercises are listed specifically in this chapter because of their ease of performance, muscle targeting, and enjoyment level. However, you should feel free to examine and use the moves listed in other chapters as well as long as you keep in mind proper technique and safety. Chapter Four: The Facts About Resistance Training for Women and Chapter Five: The Facts About Resistance Training for Men specifically list other free weight exercises. These are best done with a trainer until the correct form is mastered.

Farmer's Walk

Place a dumbbell in each hand. Rise up on your toes. This is a cool exercise to do around a mat because the mat gives you a designated perimeter. A basketball circle is another good choice. While on your toes, walk around your designated path. This is really going to work your calves so don't overdo it. It's also working your shoulders, your abs, and so on. Your balance is being tested and trained.

Single Dumbbell Deadlift Squat

If you've read the sections on Women's and Men's Resistance Training (Chapters Four and Five respectively) then you know I'm a big fan of the deadlift/squat/bench press combination. The Single Dumbbell Deadlift Squat move combines two of those moves for a powerful workout that hits major muscles including your abs and back, quads and hamstrings, and, of course, your glutes, and your calves. Because you're holding the dumbbell in your bent arms, you're also working your biceps, triceps, and forearms a bit. That's a lot of muscles.

Start with a wide-leg stance, slightly wider than shoulder-width and the dumbbell gripped in both hands hanging down in front of you. You are standing in a straight, powerful posture with your abdominals engaged. Lower yourself to a squat with the dumbbell between your knees. Keep your chest up. Push through the floor and squeeze your glutes as you give a powerful push up to a stand. That is one completed rep. Repeat about 6 times for a set.

See-Saw Row

We are going to use pretty light weights for this. Hold one dumbbell in each hand. Bend at the waist to a comfortable position. Keeping your back straight and elbows in, alternately pull up one elbow to above the back then, while lowering it, raise the other. Continue to alternate for allotted repetitions.

Lying Chest Press

Lying on the mat, a dumbbell in each hand, elbows out to the side, raise your arms to full extension directly above the chest. Bring arms gently back to the ground just barely touching down before rising back up again.

Overhead Tricep Extension

One dumbbell is all that's needed. Put the weight behind and over your head with your elbows in. Bending just your elbows, lower and extend the weight. Be sure to keep the weight evenly balanced between both arms so both arms are working equally.

Alternating Dumbbell Curls

One dumbbell in each hand, hands at your sides. For this move, you will bend your arms to curl the dumbbell to your shoulder, swiveling your pinky towards your chest, thus, working your bicep. Do not use momentum to swing the dumbbell up. Do not swivel shoulders or hips. This is a relatively still move that should isolate your arms and be done slowly and controlled unless you are performing a burnout.

Weight Machines

Weight machines are generally designed for the long limbs of a full-grown adult so they will not be appropriate for most growing athletes. However, if you are one of those exceptional students who are adult-sized before you're full-grown, then weight machines are a possibility for you. Your gym will teach you the basics of using its equipment with your introductory membership. Be sure to always use proper technique. One advantage of weight machines is that it is more difficult to go awry with technique than if you are using free weights or even resistance bands for resistance training.

If you are of a full-grown height so that you can accommodate the weight machines properly, please refer to one of the other chapters for suggested exercises. See Chapter Four: The Facts About Resistance Training for Women and Chapter Five: The Facts About Resistance Training for Men.

Apply the same starting weight rules that you applied for free weights: if you can do ten repetitions with the last two being increasingly difficult, you're at the right weight.

NOTE: When doing these forms of exercises proceed step by step, don't over do it and if you have been able to do 10 preps of press-ups a day, don't jump to doing 50 preps.

Be careful with the weight machines. Lifting more than your body can sustain can lead to an injury. Pay close attention to your body and if you feel a lot of pain during the weight lifts, please stop the weights.

CHAPTER SEVEN: WHY IS THERE SO MUCH BAD PRESS ON RESISTANCE TRAINING?

"Myth vs Reality"

The popular myth that resistance training was not only potentially harmful to young athletes but was also of little use for improving strength and power was first fostered in the research community. One of the earliest forms of research came from Eastern Europe back in the early 1960s. A study investigating the trainability of lower back muscles following a course of isometric resistance training failed to demonstrate any significant improvements in strength.

In recent years, research has started to provide compelling evidence of the benefits of resistance training.

Although testosterone is responsible for strength and muscle growth, young boys can also experience gains in strength.

So how can children improve strength if testosterone is not responsible? Testosterone does not start to increase until mid to late puberty, effectively ruling out the male hormone's contribution to strength gains in young athletes. Given those adolescent girls, and women in general, hardly produce any testosterone (maybe 1/16th at best) compared to boys, young girls, and women who improve their muscular strength point in the direction of a different explanation.

Evidence suggests that strength increases in line with the development of the nervous system, which is of primary importance in the exertion and development of muscular strength. Research has indicated that there are three likely determinants of strength gains: improved motor skill coordination, increased motor unit activation, and undetermined neurological adaptations.

Can you really swim faster, jump higher and hit harder?

In short, 'YES'. While you may be prepared to accept the body of laboratory evidence which shows that resistance training can improve strength in young athletes and that the dominant underlying mechanism is neural in origin, it is legitimate to ask whether this can be translated to the sporting arena.

Sports such as soccer, football, martial arts (TaeKwonDo or Judo), tennis and track and field all require strength and power in order to perform complex multi-joint movements. It's not unreasonable, based on the research, to suggest that the results seen in controlled laboratory studies could be transferred to the sporting arena. Although there is limited direct research in this area, some data have shown that intensive resistance training can improve both speed and power in pre-adolescent boys and girls.

But what about injuries? Surely, all that training can't be good for young bodies?

In 1987, the U. S. Consumer Product Safety Commission reported that resistance training was a harmful activity for children. The report highlighted the disturbingly large number of injuries associated with resistance-type exercises: 8,543 injuries were incurred by 0 to 14-year-olds and ranged in severity from sprains and strains to fractures. Approximately 40% of the injuries occurred during unsupervised sessions in the home. A subsequent study, investigating sport-related injuries in school children taking part in 22 sports, found that resistance training produced just seven injuries from a total of 637, placing it 17th on the injurious list.

But what about the immature musculoskeletal system?

Another area of concern is the potential damage resistance training can cause to the immature skeleton: increased physical activity in children is often associated with musculoskeletal damage. The skeletal system is in its formative stages during preadolescence and does not fully mature until early adulthood. It is commonly thought that the use of resistance training could contribute to damage of cartilage, bones, joint surfaces, and tendons. It has even been suggested that damage to growth cartilage can result in stunted growth. Note: that's why parents enroll their kids in programs like martial arts, yoga, gymnastics - to help increase strength and flexibility.

I personally like the myth that if a child or young athlete starts performing resistance squatting movements too soon they may fuse their lower back vertebrae together. I mean, let's use some common sense here, and check with your physician first, but any fracture of the vertebrae wouldn't just stunt their growth. *It would put them in a wheelchair as well!* Honestly, in all my years of weight training, I've never seen this happen. EVER!

Other structures, such as the spine, have also been highlighted as an area of potential injury. Although these issues are a serious cause for concern, some experts feel that the case may be somewhat overstated. Research has shown that sport-related musculoskeletal damage occurs very rarely. The majority of cases have been linked with maximal over-head lifts of the sort associated with powerlifting, and no evidence has been found of skeletal damage in relation to resistance training.

Or what about the myth of converting fat into muscle? With the knowledge presented in this text, I'm sure you realize that fat and muscle are two different biological compounds and structures in the body. From a scientific standpoint that would be like converting *milk* to *orange juice*! In fact, if you're losing weight and not eating enough protein, the body will burn the *muscle* as well as the fat. It doesn't differentiate between tissues, it just needs fuel. If there's no protein for fuel, it burns whatever tissue it can find - be it fat *or* muscle. So diet is essential.

That means a good mix of proteins, carbohydrates, and fats with enough vitamins and minerals to stay healthy. Minimize added sugars. But that doesn't mean you can't indulge in ice cream now and then - just make it a small one. Stay away from processed foods as much as possible. When it comes to carbohydrates like bread, rice, and pasta, opt for the whole grain kinds whenever possible. And finally, a minimum of salt. Most of our foods today come with added salt and we really don't need much at all to stay healthy, so minimize any addition of it to keep it as low as possible to avoid an increase in blood pressure, heart disease and stroke.

Resistance training will not turn the obese person into a muscle machine. But a combination of diet and exercise will help you lose fat and resistance training can be an excellent part of an exercise program that will strengthen bones and muscles contributing to improved self-esteem and self-confidence which will encourage continued participation in physical activities.

Some people think resistance training is a bad idea because muscle means bulk and bulk slows you down. Muscle doesn't have to mean bulk. And it certainly doesn't mean slowing down. Here are some of the crazy things you might read on the internet that people say:

"Despite the ability to stay fast with weights, it does still slow you down. The more muscle you gain, the more oxygen your body uses, thus requiring even more cardio." - anonymous quote from the internet.

"I was an in and out volume fighter (think Cuban fighters in Olympics)- the amount of cardio I needed was very high. The oxygen that would have been required had I put on more muscle would have been a disservice to me for sure. - ShamrockAPD"

"Big muscles are somewhat counterproductive when it comes to fighting. Combat sports are all about speed, agility, and stamina. Big muscles tend to diminish all of those. Harder to throw faster, less flexible, and being heavier tires you out faster".

It's comments like these all over the internet that leave people thinking that weight training is somehow bad for or goes against techniques needed for MMA, boxing, and combat fighting. Finally, an intelligent one:

"Because a lot of people still believe that lifting weights will make you gain weight and get too slow. It can, but it doesn't have to. I started lifting, and I'm the same weight, I'm just as fast, but my power has gone up. Rep ranges, frequency of lifting, and caloric intake will affect your weight. - dirt_shitters"

While it's true that extra muscle can move your weight into a heavier class, it doesn't have to. Remember, the training we're talking about here is not about BULK. It's about STRENGTH. And every fighter needs strength. Every bit of fighting requires strength, from throwing a punch to grappling. You're not gonna throw a roundhouse kick if you're not strong and resistance training gives you strength.

Brett Jones (center for the Minnesota Vikings football team) said, "Absolute strength is the glass. Everything else is the liquid inside the glass. The bigger the glass, the more of everything else you can do." Meaning, you must have the strength to do anything.

How do you get strength without the bulk? Your central nervous system fires up many little motor units that make up one muscle. It responds best to high intensity for low volume. That means higher weight for fewer repetitions with longer rest periods between. Similar to the HIIT workouts we've already talked about. Because all the muscles are connected to the little motors connected to the nervous system, we're essentially training the nervous system when we exercise. If we use a little trick called hyper-irradiation, we recruit many muscles at once to train the nervous system into engaging them all each time you use one or more.

A prime example of hyper-irradiation is used when you are performing any of our three core free weight moves that work to make up an essential full-body routine. When you bench press, rather than engaging just the chest and arms, you engage all those other muscles as well: deltoids, biceps, triceps, quads, abs, and so on. Same with squats. Not just your target muscle - the glutes, but all the muscles engageable: abs, hamstrings, quads, calves, all of it. The deadlift is no exception. Yes, you'll engage your trapezius, latissimus dorsi, and teres major (these are the major back muscles, in case you didn't pick up on that). But you'll also engage all the other muscles you can possibly involve including deltoids, flexors, triceps brachii, vastus lateralis (one of the back of the thigh muscles), biceps femoris (the other back of the thigh muscle), and on down the body.

When you're powerful like this, an opponent trying to knock you off your feet has a much more difficult time because all of your muscles connected to your stance - even if you don't think they are - are firing at once because you taught your nervous system to do that with this training. That includes the little muscles in your neck which are part of a stable back. Bet you didn't know that.

To build this kind of strength, without building muscle, we'll do the maximal lifting. (See chapter 8 for restrictions to these moves.) That means a heavy weight (60% of 1 rep max) moved as fast as possible (with complete control) to activate as many fast-twitch muscles as possible. That's where our power three moves come in again because they activate so many muscles. What are those three big, basic, important moves again? Bench press, deadlift, and squats.

Lift explosively. Here are some exercises to try:

Wood Choppers

This can be done with a kettlebell, a dumbbell, or a cable. The following are instructions for kettlebell or dumbbell. The move is the same for both - when you move to a cable, you will need to step further from the stack to keep the weights from touching down between moves and you will be pulling from the waist. You are going to use an oblique twist with a burst of power. Stand with your feet slightly wider than hip-width apart. Swivel on your left foot as you raise your weight up above head height to the right in a firm controlled grip. Swing down hard to the left as you lower into a squat bringing the ball to the outside of your knee. Swing the ball back up to the right pivoting on the ball of your left foot. Repeat on the other side.

Frog Jumps

Lower yourself into a ¾ squat. You will push up from the ground launching yourself into the air with a forward tilt as your arms swing forward for momentum. Think distance. Land softly by bending your knees to absorb the impact while your arms swing back to your sides.

Clean & Jerk

This move improves shoulder and hip mobility and stability. This is another power move that covers a vast majority of muscles from your calves all the way up to your trapezius brachii and absolutely every muscle in between. It covers all of those beautiful abdominal muscles: rectus abdominis, serratus, and external obliques. It rocks your back: infraspinatus, trapezius, and latissimus Dorsi on down into your gluteus maximus. This move powers your abductors, semitendinosus (little muscle on the back of your thigh just above the calf), both your calf muscles (gastrocnemius lateral head and medial head), and I haven't yet mentioned what it does for your arms. Both the biceps and triceps brachii get worked along with your deltoids (shoulders). Of course, your chest (pectoralis major) and your lats (latissimus dorsi - those great muscles that give you 'wings') get shredded with this move too.

Now let's learn how to do it.

There are two moves here. The first brings the bar to your chest. The second jerks it overhead. Grasp the bar bent over from a shoulder-width leg stance. Pull the bar to your waist then dip your knees to jerk it up to your chest in a squat move. Now you will explode your force upwards thrusting the bar overhead often with a split leg position. Bring back down by touching the bar briefly to the chest, the hips, and then lowering to the floor.

Medicine Ball Throws

There are lots of ways to throw a medicine ball. And they're all right! Here are a few to get you started with explosive, power generating, *fun* throws to try.

- Underhand throw
- Remember granny throws from basketball? Same idea.
- Take the ball in both hands
- Squat with it between your knees
- Toss the ball as high as you can and catch it.
- Reverse Throw - for this exercise, you will need a less dense medicine ball that will bounce slightly.
- Throw the ball up and behind you
- Swivel to catch it on the bounce
- Side Toss

- Toss it to the side with a two-hand toss for rotational power.
- Scurry to the side to catch.
- This can also be done against a wall.
- Shot Put Throw
- This is great with a partner or even against a wall. Or…do the running to follow after the ball
- Hold the ball in one hand, swivel-throw it as though you were throwing a shot put, pushing it past your face and out into the air on the opposite side of your body.
- Sit Up Throw
- Need to get off the mat fast? As in grappling? Or if you fall in soccer and need to quickly scurry up to follow the ball? This move helps with the muscles involved in that.
- Lay flat on your back with knees bent, medicine ball in your hands stretched out past your head.
- Explode your arms upward as you sit up and throw the ball forward.
- A good one to do with a partner who can return the ball to you.

Kettlebell Swings

This begins in a deadlift position, only you're holding a kettlebell instead of a bar. Get a good grip on the kettlebell. Your next move is to swing the weight between your legs then explode it up to chest height where you are in a tightened core, standing plank position. Explode your breath in an exhale as you bring that bell to a stop at your chest. Arc it back down. You must maintain control of the kettlebell at all times. Bend your knees but do not squat.

The explosiveness of these moves is great for building strong muscles without adding bulk. They light up all the fast-twitch muscles in use making them ready to burst into action when they're needed - in a martial arts bout, boxing, or whatever your chosen sport.

CHAPTER EIGHT: THE TRAINING SYSTEMS

"Finding the Right Training Program for You."

There are many states you need to be focused on as training goals. When you start training in any exercise activity, you will want a specific result, either weight loss, muscle building, or cardiovascular fitness. Most of the time you would want a combination of all three results. Each type of training involves different techniques, exercises, and often, pieces of equipment. I will do my best to explain each system in detail.

A 'rep,' or 'repetition,' is an exercise movement performed by lifting a weight from the start, to the top of the movement, and back down again. A series of single repetitions done in succession and then terminated is called a 'set.' Exercise routines are traditionally composed of combinations of sets and reps. Other variations of sets and reps include partial range reps, isometric reps (no movement), and peak contraction reps (squeezing a muscle at the top). All of these elements have a place in a well-rounded training regimen.

Sets can become more elaborate, also. A superset is when a trainee performs two sets for the same or different muscles, without resting in between them. Tri-sets are three sets performed in a row with no rest. Circuit training is one *giant set* performed with no rest at all until the prescribed number of sets is complete.

These terms are specific to the training goals that follow.

The young athlete:

a) should complete a medical examination by a qualified physician before starting any training program

b) he/she should be mature enough to accept instruction

c) should want to participate in the program

d) must possess the basic motor skills of their primary sport

e) must maintain correct form during lifting

f) must avoid competition during training

The instructor or trainer should:

a) ensure the young athlete is closely supervised during training sessions

b) ensure the training offers variety (to avoid boredom and drop out)

c) pay particular attention to the strengthening of the back and abdominal muscles

d) ensure that in the event of any pain, training is discontinued

d) ensure that the resistance training program forms part of a comprehensive program designed to increase motor skills and fitness levels

e) ensure that all exercises are carried out through a full range of motion (ROM)

f) Prohibit any attempts at maximal lifts. (Hint: for more natural results, have the young athletes perform resistance exercises using their own body weight. This will build up their natural strength first before they start performing routines on machines.)

g) Start your circuit training program on exercise equipment and machines first then work your way to free weights. Advantages: For beginners, the equipment balances the weight load for you, leaving you to concentrate on the exercised body part. Additionally, there is less chance of improper technique because the machine only allows for a certain degree of movement.

BASIC RESISTANCE TRAINING GUIDELINES

If resistance training is a new area for you, here are some of the basic guidelines you should think of when putting together a training program:

1. Begin and end each session with 5-10 minutes of warm-up and stretching.
2. Balance the workout by altering pairs of muscle groups, i.e. perform a 'pull' exercise after each 'push' exercise.
   (Examples of pull exercises are barbell or dumbbell bent-over row, cable lat. pulldown, seated row; push exercises may include barbell, dumbbell or machine bench press, squats, and shoulder press.)
3. Exercise the larger muscle groups (pectoralis major - chest; latissimus dorsi -back; quadriceps) first, and the smaller muscle groups (biceps and triceps - arms; deltoids - shoulder; gastrocnemius/soleus - calves) at the end.
4. Perform 1 to 3 sets of 6 to 15 repetitions. Younger children may use fewer sets and more repetitions.
5. Allow 48 hours of recovery after each strength training session.
6. Work on the schedule 2 to 3 times per week while maintaining other sporting activities.

7. Younger children can spend 20 to 30 minutes per session while older children can increase the duration of each session.

Determining Starting Weight

A good starting weight is one that you can easily lift ten times with the last two repetitions becoming more and more difficult. When those two are also easy, increase your weight. If you struggle to get to ten, you need to lower down your weight to something lighter.

Motivation

What's going to get you to the gym or the track or wherever it is you workout and get you moving? Most of the time, it will simply be your inner desire to succeed in your chosen sport, be that martial arts, MMA, boxing, combat fighting of any kind, or any other individual or team competition. Sometimes, you'll be working out just to improve your physical well-being. But there will be days when the desire just is not there. What then?

You need a motivator. Whether you feel like it or not, get yourself to the gym. As you're working your way through the easy stuff - the joint rolls and quick bout of aerobics that make up your warm-up, and into your stretches, focus your mind on one of these motivators.

- Promise yourself an after workout reward. Such as a round of your favorite video game when you've successfully completed your workout. Or put a dollar in a jar for every workout and when you've made enough, splurge on that big reward you've wanted. Maybe it's a weight set for home. Or your own resistance bands. Or a membership at a really fine gym. Whatever it is, go for it - you earned it! How 'bout a slick new pair of kicks? Or the new fitness tracker everyone's been talking about. Anything fitness related is an excellent, double-duty motivator.
- When you need to put on that last little bit of stamina to

finish your burn out, imagine a Tyrannosaurus Rex chasing after you. If you don't run as fast as you can, you'll be his dinner.

- Remember Rocky Balboa. How many times did he get back up after being beaten down? Not just by opponents, but by life itself. Imagine you're him, riding the eye of the tiger, racing up those steps toward the Art Museum. You can do it.

- Give yourself five minutes. Plug through your warm-up and stretches - the easy part which takes little to no effort. Now you're ready for the workout. At that point, set an alarm for five minutes. If, when it goes off, you still just don't feel like you can do any more work, you have full permission to skip today. Chances are, though, you will be ready to move forward, to keep plowing through what you've already started. After all, T-Rex is on your tail!

- We've talked numerous times about changing up your routine. Maybe the change you need is not in the exercises but rather in the location. Try a new park for your run. Or workout inside instead of outside or vice versa. Or use a trial membership at a new gym for a change of scenery. You're not cheating. You'll return to old faithful. You're just taking a change of scene.

- Maybe it's time to get competitive. Competing isn't for everyone. But it just may be the motivating factor you've been looking for. Working towards a goal like a competition can be highly motivating. If this is something you'd like to do, consult with your trainer to make a plan to choose the appropriate competition, set up a workout that progresses you towards winning that competition, and begin your training. Nothing can be more motivating than the goal of a big win.

- Money can be a big motivator. Getting your money's worth out of your gym membership can be a reason to get there and workout. All that money you're spending to be a member of your favorite gym, see if you can work out enough times to keep the cost under $20/visit.

- Put your money in a private trainer. You're getting someone who's expecting you to be there for every workout - a motivator in itself - plus you're spending your hard-earned money on each and every workout so you want to get the most out of it you possibly can. That means working your hardest. Motivation enough?

- Think positive. Think of all the great reasons you have for working out. You'll be healthier, stronger. You'll look great! Think "I'll look great at the beach!" Or "I'll be able to climb all the way to the top of the mountain." Think of the end result that you're producing to help motivate you through today's workout.

- Use what you see. Like the new and improved you after just a short time working out? Post that picture up where you can see it to help you want to make even more improvements. Or maybe you only need the motivation of knowing a good girl (boy, woman, man) is waiting for you. Post their picture up to remind you that you're getting fit to make the times with them even more pleasurable. Or, if you are headed to the beach/mountains/whitewater rafting, post up a picture of that to keep your eyes on the prize and your motivation at full tilt.

- Motivation is what gets you started. Habit is what keeps you going. So all you need is the motivation to get to the gym.

- When you're about to quit - or fail to get started today - remember why you started working out in the first place. Was it to lose weight? To build up some muscle? To compete? Whatever the original motivator, focus on that thought, focus on that original motivator, pull it up from inside of you, and use it again. Get up and get moving.

- Focus on the outcome. Don't think about this moment of effort or pain. Focus instead on the finish, the success.

- Visualization: If T-Rex didn't do it for you, try this: WWII in the Aleutian Islands, it was bitter cold, and wet. Fingers could barely bend to hang on to wrenches. But the ground crew had to battle the freezing rain and mid-calf deep mud to prepare the planes for the next squadron to take off. The whole world depended on it. If they could fight that battle - and win - then you can battle a chilly morning run, a hot afternoon resistance training, a rain-soaked end of workout burn out. Neither rain, nor sleet, nor snow, nor dark of night (Ok, that's the post office. But it still applies.) will keep you from reaching your goal. Fight it out. And win! It's just a little weather.

And now for some fighting words. Anyone of these should motivate you to keep at it:

- The only disability in life is a bad attitude.
- When you're about to quit, remember why you started.
- A little sweat ain't never hurt nobody.
- When I'm dripping with sweat, I feel badass.
- Train like a beast, look like a beauty.
- A champion is someone who gets up when they can't.
- Nothing's over until you stop trying.
- Wake up. Work out. Look hot. Kick ass.
- The real workout starts when you want to stop.
- Better sore than sorry.
- It's not swagger, I'm just sore.
- I'm doing this for me.
- You've got what it takes, but it will take everything you've got.
- No matter how slow you go, you're still lapping everybody on the couch.
- Someone who is busier than you is running right now.
- Yes, I killed it. But I'm just getting started.
- I might not be perfect, but, damn, I'm progressing.
- You have a choice: you can throw in the towel, or you can use it to wipe the sweat off your face.

- You don't *have* to do this; you *get* to do this.
- Tough times don't last. Tough people do.
- I workout because some part of me still believes I can be… *Xena Warrior Princess* (fill in your own superhero. LOL. This one's taken.)
- The only one who can beat me is me.
- Be stronger than your excuses.
- Skinny girls look good in clothes. Fit girls look good naked.
- The most critical decision is made when you feel like giving up.
- Make your body the sexiest outfit you own.
- If you give up now, then what was the point of everything.
- Don't dream of it - train for it!
- Of course, it's hard. It's supposed to be hard. If it were easy, everybody would do it. Hard is what makes it great. - *A-League of Their Own*
- Today be the badass you were too lazy to be yesterday.
- Good things come to those who sweat.
- Once you see results, it becomes an addiction.
- A tiger doesn't lose sleep over the opinion of sheep.

Wow! That just motivated me right out of my chair. You folks will have to wait till after my workout to get any more. I'm outta her

CHAPTER NINE: NATURAL WEIGHT (BODYWEIGHT) TRAINING ROUTINES

"Some of my Favorites see if it works for You"

Natural weight training is the key to maintaining your flexibility and mobility no matter your age and fitness level. Bodyweight training enables you to utilize your muscle group, burn tons of calories, and improve your heart rate health. It is considered one of the best methods of burning calories within a short period of time.

Young individuals have an improved performance because their body undergoes hormonal changes and other physiological changes that enable them to maximize their strength, build muscle mass, and improve their athletic performance.

You don't have to spend hours in the gym for you to obtain the desired results. You can easily do the workouts at home in a few simple steps. In today's corporate world, a lot of people don't have enough time to go to the gym and workout. So these training routines will help busy and time-challenged individuals to easily improve their health and be able to feel better after a stressful day.

We have collected some of the best bodyweight exercises that you can use whenever and wherever so as to build your strength and have a lean body. Ready to feel better, grab your towel and let me guide you through an efficient bodyweight routine.

WHAT IS A BODYWEIGHT EXERCISE?

A bodyweight exercise is a form of exercise that involves movement of your bodyweight only. It is a strength training exercise that depends on the individual's weight to provide the required resistance against gravity. The bodyweight exercises are an effective way to enhance your balance, strength, power, speed, endurance, and flexibility without using any gym equipment.

These exercises involve jumping, pushing, pulling, or doing an activity that relies on your body weight as resistance alone.

Bodyweight training offers a lot of benefits to individuals of all ages. So why should you get into bodyweight training exercises?

1. Convenience

With bodyweight training, you require little or no equipment. You only need your sportswear and you're good to go. There is no time wasted going to and from your gym. The exercises can also be done in your living room, basement, or in your backyard. This makes it a convenient way to do your workouts as well as maximize your time.

2. Help boost your mobility and stability

Your mobility and stability are an important part of your life. When doing movements during bodyweight training, you will be able to increase your mobility and boost your body's muscle stabilizers. This will help you increase your strength.

3. Suitable for everyone

Bodyweight exercises are beginner-friendly and suitable for everyone. You can implement some variations and changes to the workouts to make them incredibly challenging and interesting for you, even for the advanced weight lifters.

The workouts are great for everyone no matter your fitness level. There are always exercises for someone starting at zero and others for seasoned athletes. Keep challenging yourself for more progressive workouts since the exercises are more straightforward.

The exercises help you build your strength and you won't feel bored with your daily routine.

4. These exercises are great for preventing injuries and developing your technique

When doing weight lifting it puts a lot of stress on your joints while bodyweight training puts little stress on your joints. Therefore, you won't have any injuries that will have long-term effects on you.

Bodyweight training routines are a great way to perfect your technique and your body form. You can easily include multi-level cardio routines to your strength training exercises to make your workouts more efficient.

PRIMARY FACTORS FOR NATURAL BODYBUILDING

If you want to build your muscles, you need to take these three factors into account:

- Natural bodyweight training
- Nutrition
- Supplementation

Incorporating the right bodybuilding workouts and getting enough nutrition from your food portions will enable you desired results. If you're able to obtain all macronutrients required for a healthy body, you can skip supplementation products.

SELECTING THE BEST BODYWEIGHT WORKOUTS

Bodyweight workouts can help you gain muscle mass just as you would when lifting weights in a gym. According to published research in <u>Physiology and Behavior</u>, you can grow your muscles independently of the external load. You only need proper coordination of body movements. For example, doing squats effectively can be as great as traditional weight training methods.

As a beginner to weight training, you can't just start through countless sets of bench presses, squats, or any other type of workout. You need to rely on your body strength especially as a teen your body is still undergoing various changes.

Teenagers below the age of 14 should focus on strengthening exercises by doing basic bodyweight workouts. At this age, teens are unlikely to focus on muscle growth.

Starting with the basic workout routine will enable you to understand the best form of exercise and prepare your body to adjust gradually. In addition, it will reduce injuries that may occur if you go directly to lifting weights in a gym.

Obtaining the desired muscle growth requires you to subject your body to a lot of stress load through progressive workouts. This can easily be achieved through:

- Doing more reps in each set of workouts.
- Reducing the rest time after each set of workouts

Increasing the number of reps (times) you perform each exercise and reducing your rest time, you will be able to build lean muscles. Proper nutrition will help you repair and grow stronger muscles.

Some of the best workouts you can do at the comfort of your home include:

Set 1 workouts:

1. Basic Stretch Procedures (from top to bottom)

1. Neck Stretching

START POSITION

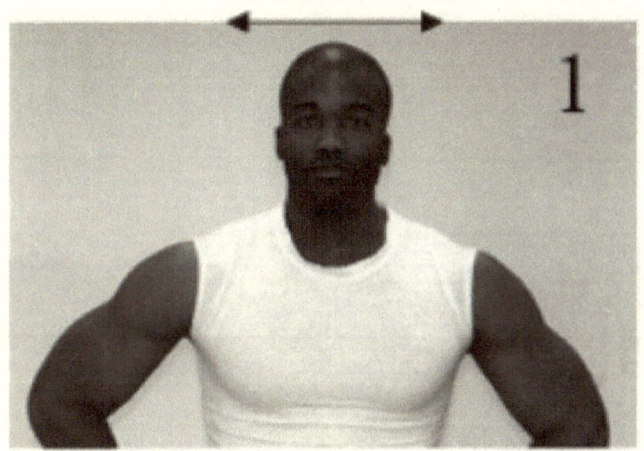

Begin by looking straight ahead.

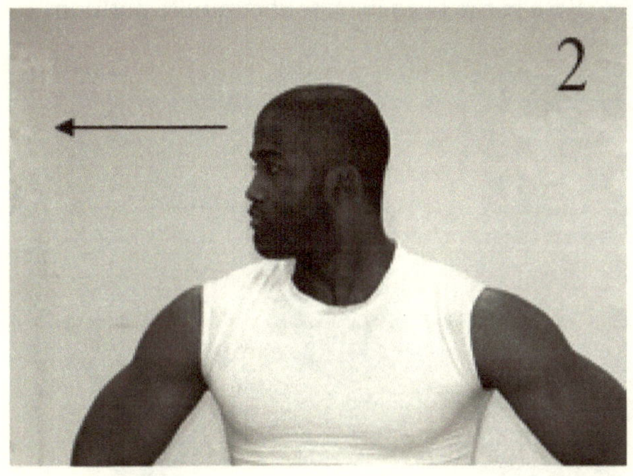

Turn the head in a natural motion to the left

MIDDLE POSITION

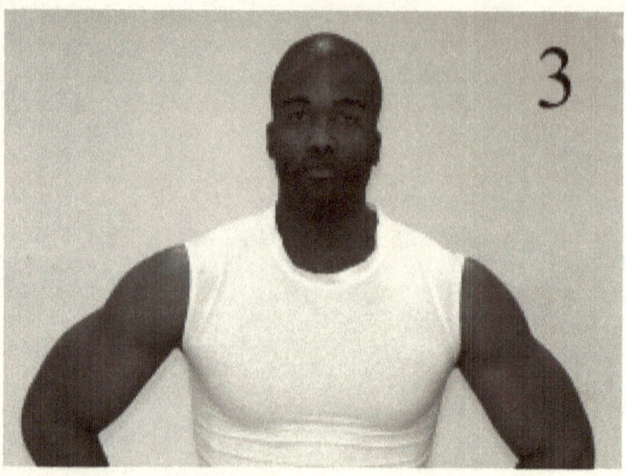

Return the head back to the middle position

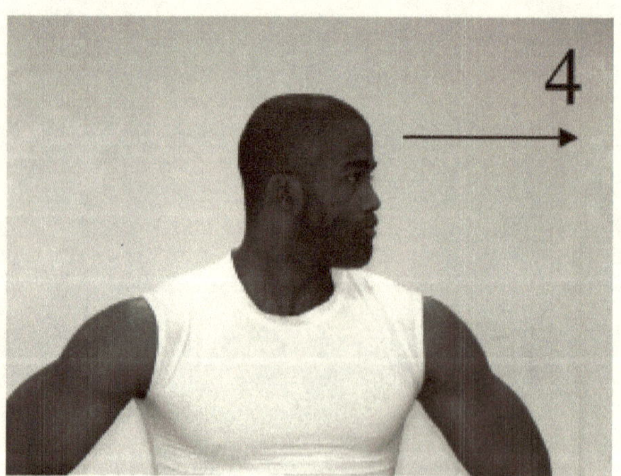

Turn the head in a natural motion to the right.

Note: This movement should be natural and without force. The whole goal is to get the head moving in a side to side motion. Try holding each position for a 10-second count.

Assisted Side Neck Stretch

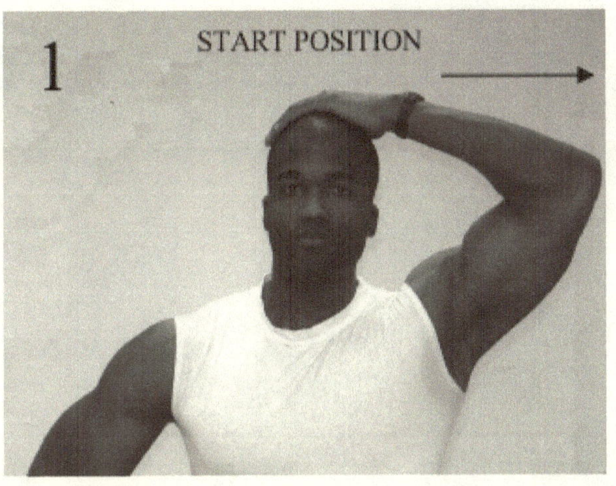

Place your hand on the top of your head

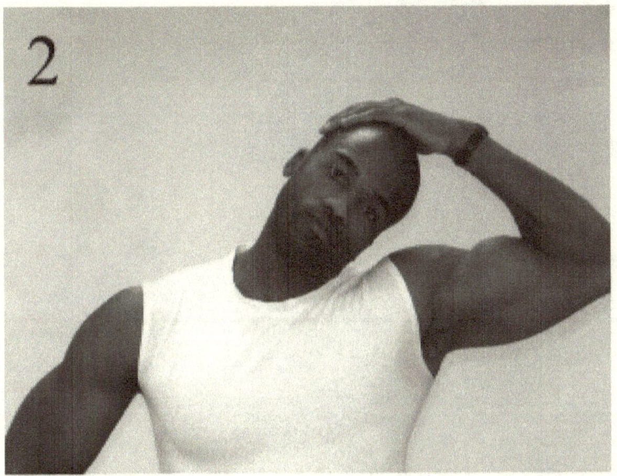

Gently pull your head down the right side.

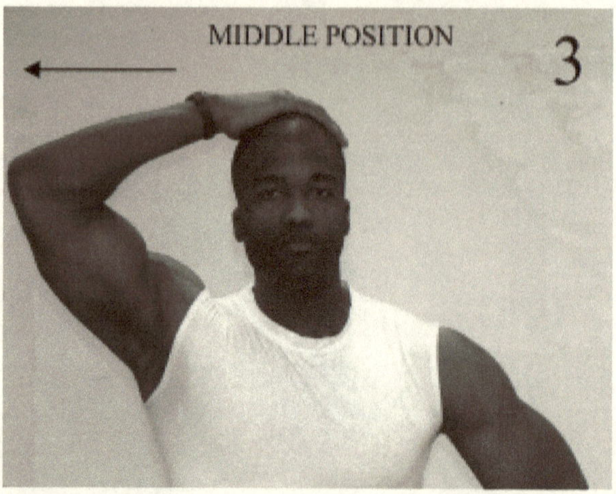

Return back to the middle position.

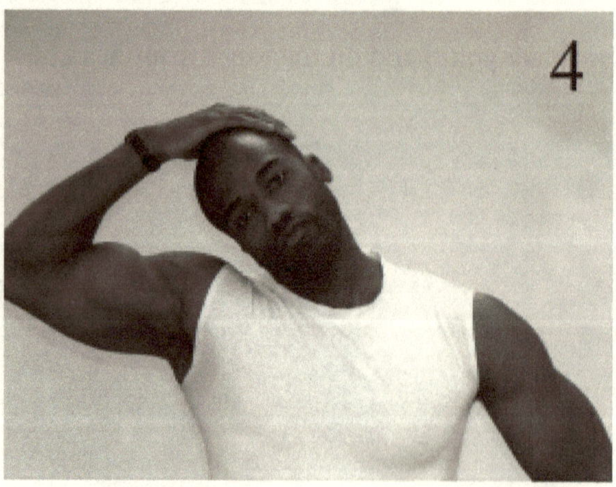

Gently pull your head down the left side.

Forward Neck Stretch

START POSITION

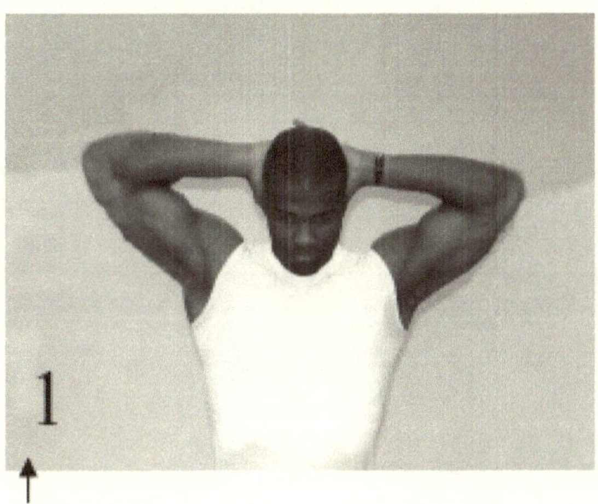

Interlock your fingers and place them both behind the neck and slowly stretch the head forward.

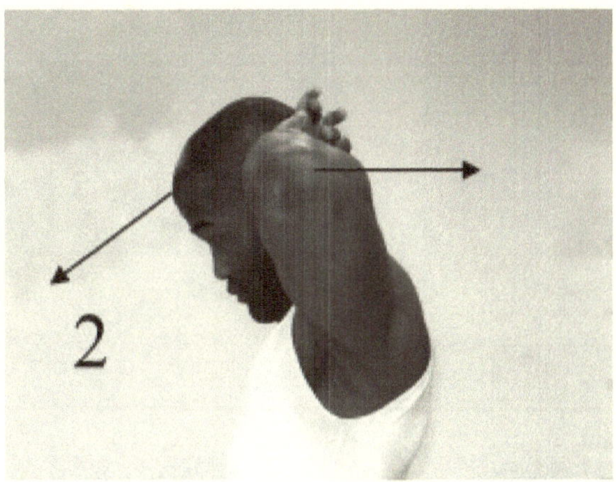

To add more pressure slowly push your elbows back!

2. Shoulder & Trunk Stretch

START _MIDDLE POSITION

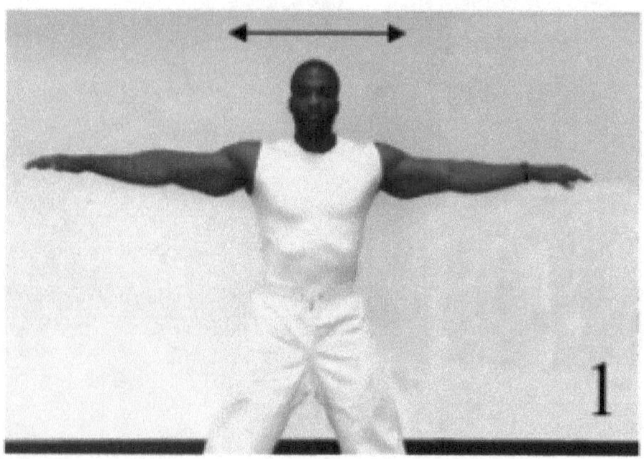

Start with both arms extended and in a straight line (180 Degrees).

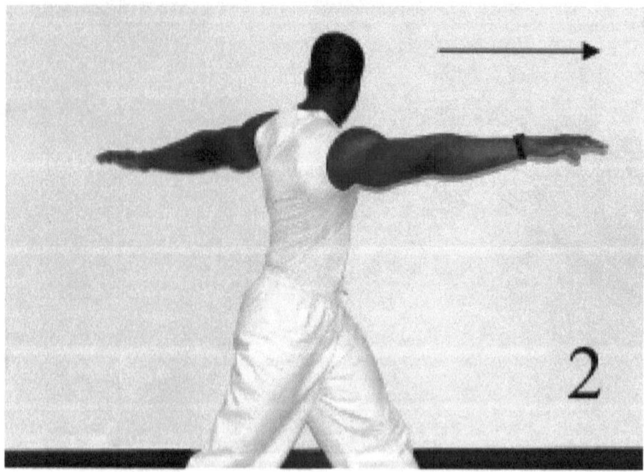

Move your right hand and twist your trunk towards the left as far as you are able to twist.

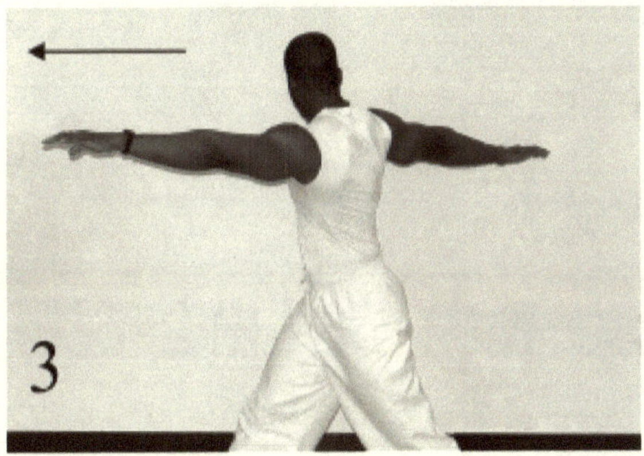

Return back to the middle position and move your left hand and twist your trunk towards the right as you are able to twist.

Note: My waist is twisting with the motion and it must be a relaxed movement and swing.

Assisted shoulder & Trunk Stretch

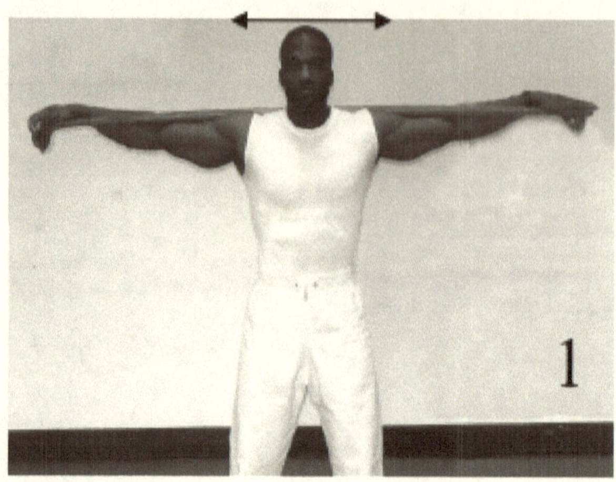

Start with both arms extended and in a straight line 180 Degrees.

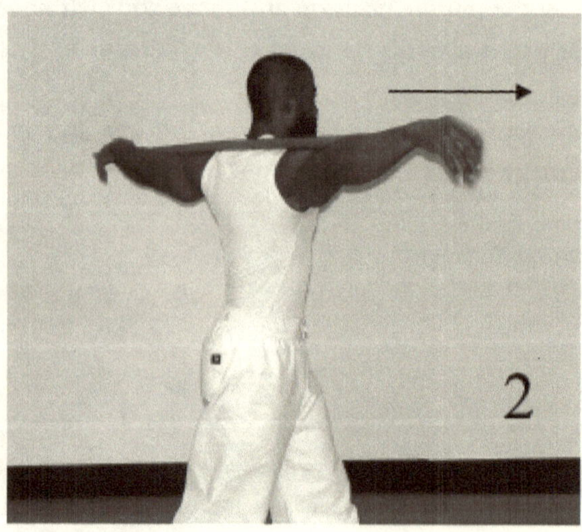

Move your right hand and twist towards the left as far as you are able to twist.

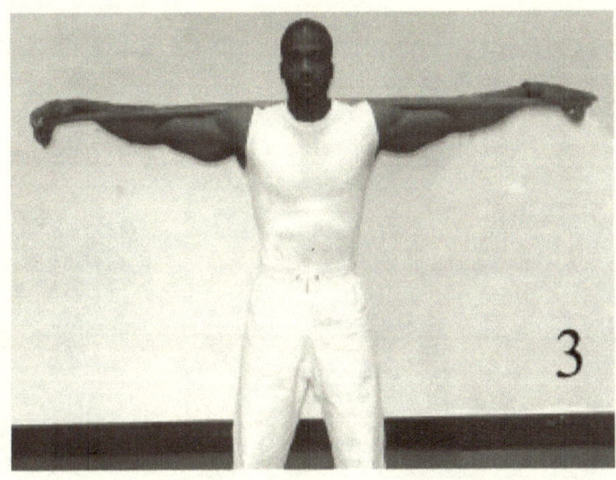

Return back to the middle position.

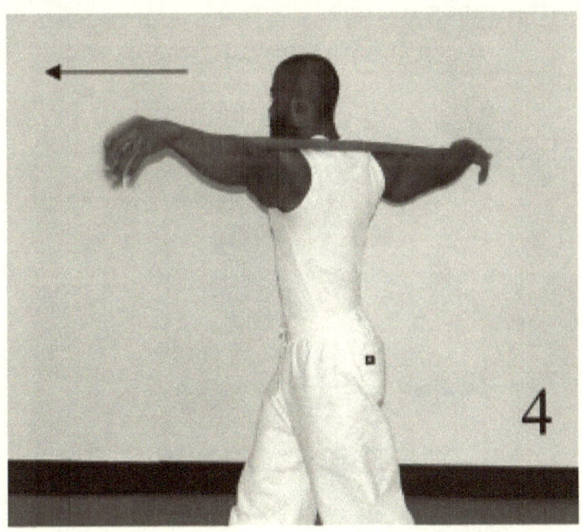

Move your left hand and twist towards the right as far as you are able to twist.

Assisted Side Shoulder Stretch

START POSITION

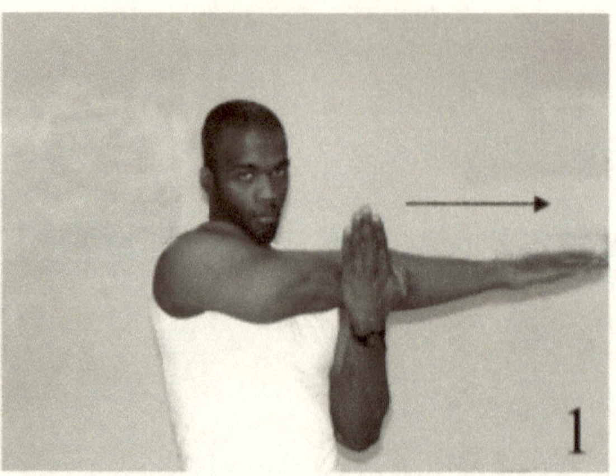

Place your left hand on the right elbow or just past it slightly towards the tricep and pull the arm towards you.

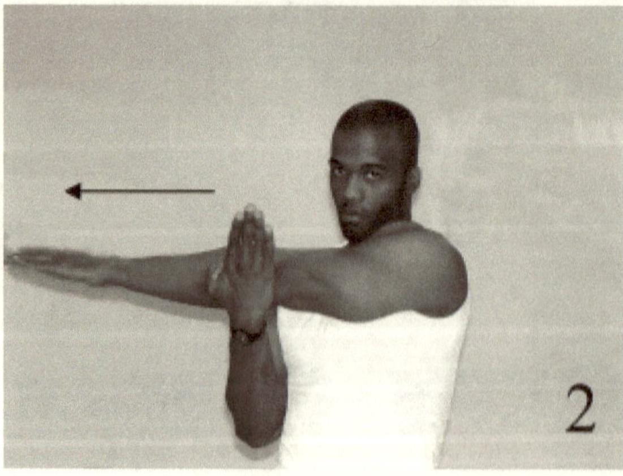

Place your right hand on your left elbow or just past it slightly towards the tricep and pull the arm towards you.

Note: When performing this stretch never pull or yank, the motion should be smooth and natural.

Shoulder Stretch

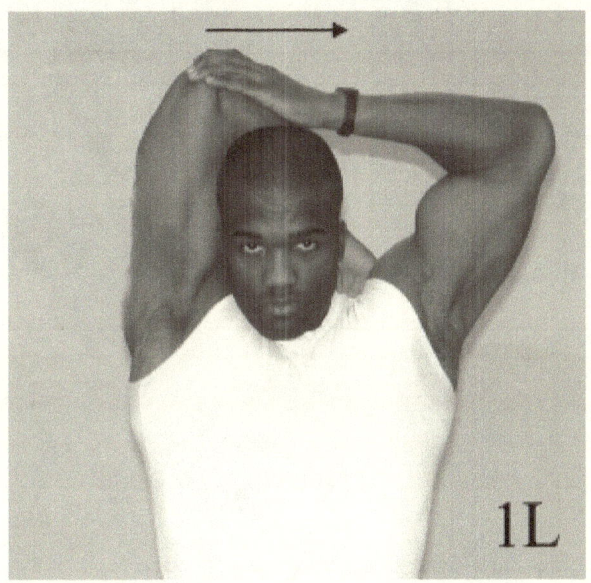

1L. Place your left arm behind your head with the elbow and slowly move the elbow towards your head. See 1BL.

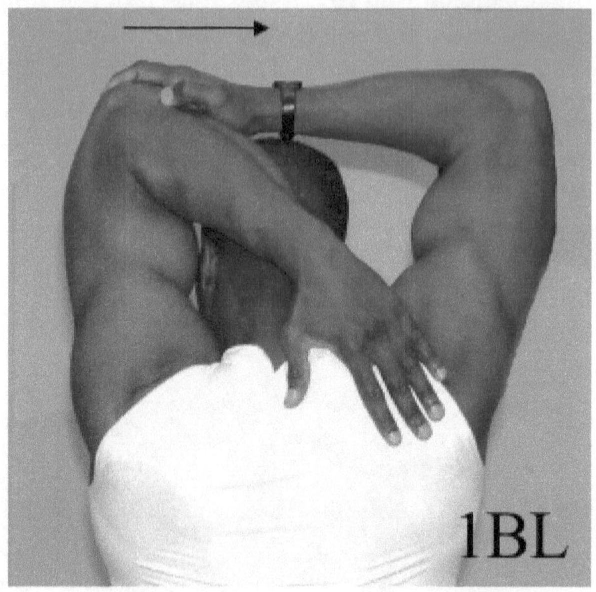

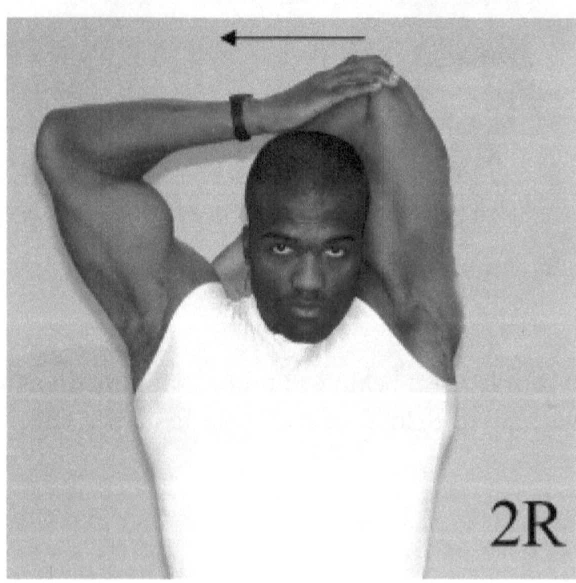

2R. Place your right arm behind your head with the elbow pointing up. Hold the raised elbow and slowly move the elbow towards your head. See 2BR.

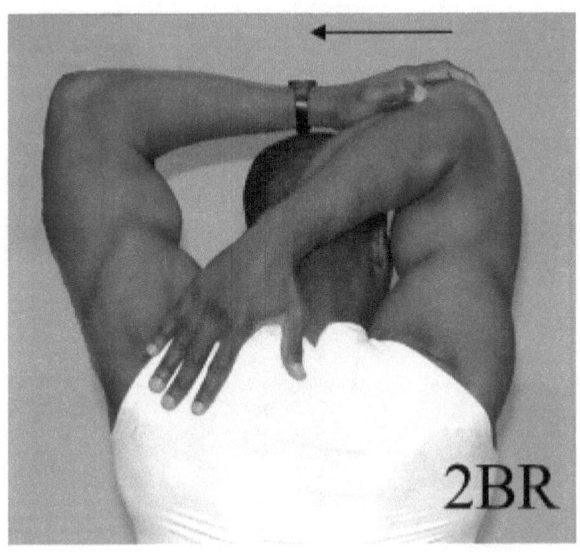

Standing Hamstring Stretch

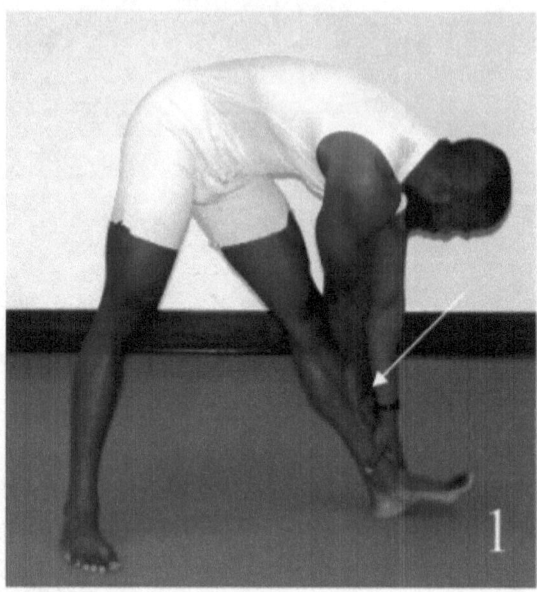

Start by taking your right foot and point the foot in 90 degrees or "L" angle. With both hands, reach down for the ankle trying to place your head on your knee.

Seating Inner Thigh and Hamstring Stretch

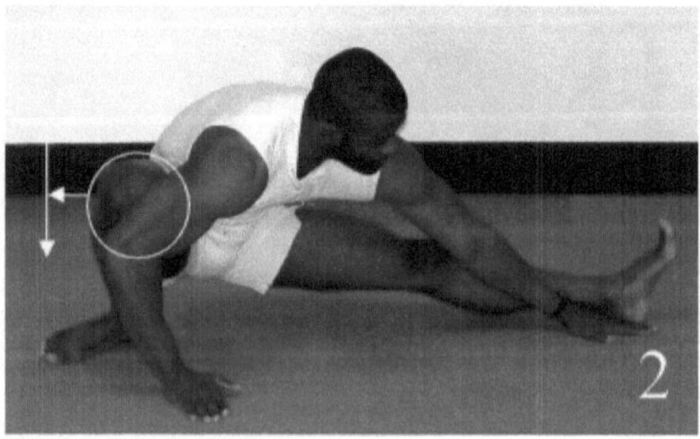

Slide the left foot out and bend the leg like a side lounge. Keep the pressure on the knee for maximum flexibility and hip ROM.

Note: My left elbow keeps that pressure on the inner part of my knee!

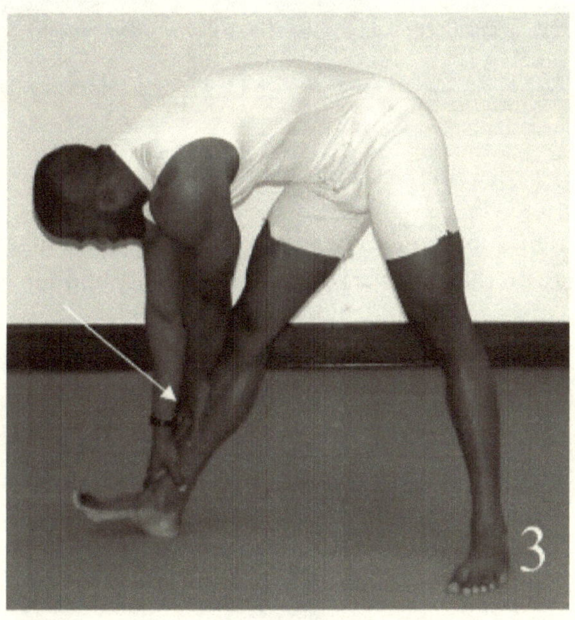

Start by taking your left foot and point the foot in 90 degrees or "L" angle. With both hands, reach down for the ankle trying to place your head to your knee.

Legs & Sitting Stretches

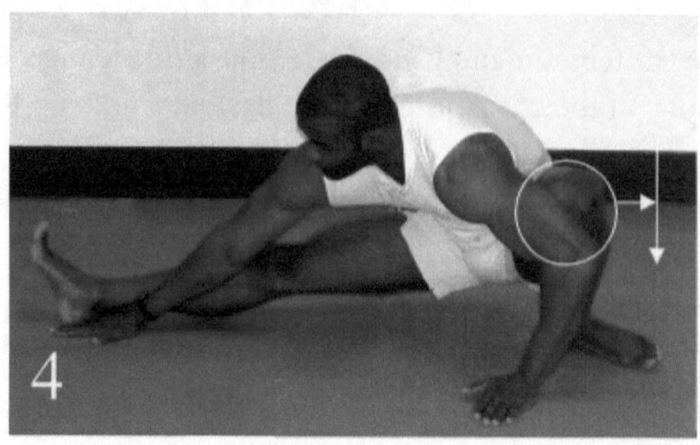

Slide the right foot out and bend the leg like a side lounge, keep the pressure on the knee for maximum flexibility and hip ROM.

Note: My right elbow keeps that pressure on the inner part of my knee!

Seated Groin or Butterfly stretch

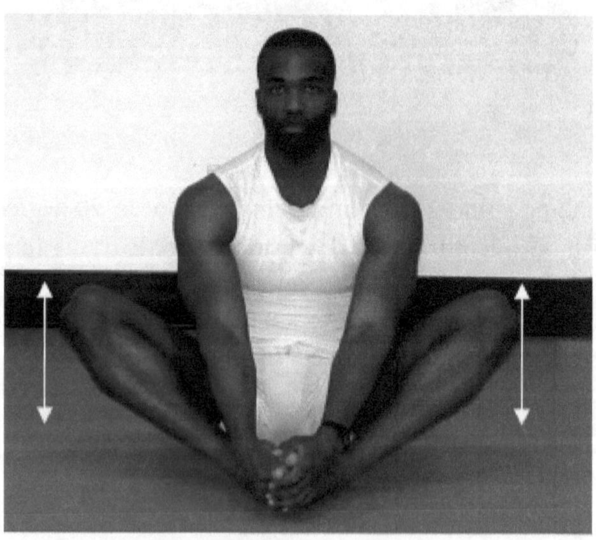

Pull both your feet into your body and hold for ten seconds. you can even do some ballistic movement (Up and Down) if you're used to this stretch position.

Note: Many Martial Arts schools have you lean forward and touch your nose to your toes or chest to the floor if you can.

Straddle Stretch

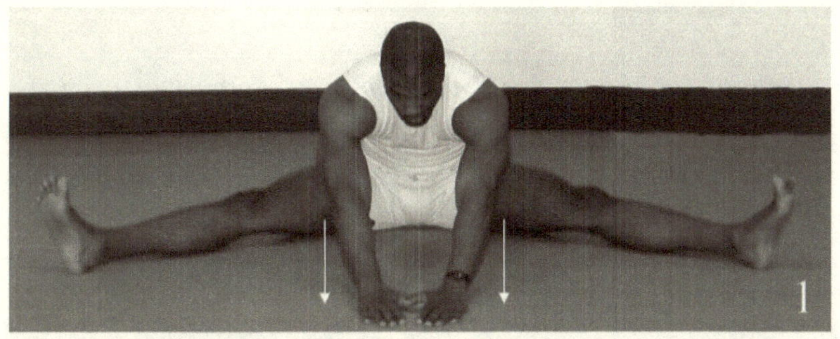

START POSITION

Start by opening your legs as far as you can go with your knees straight and your toes pointing upward. Use your hands to lean forward as far as you can go and hold for a ten-second count.

Note: If your knees start to bend, you've gone too far and the stretch is wasted.

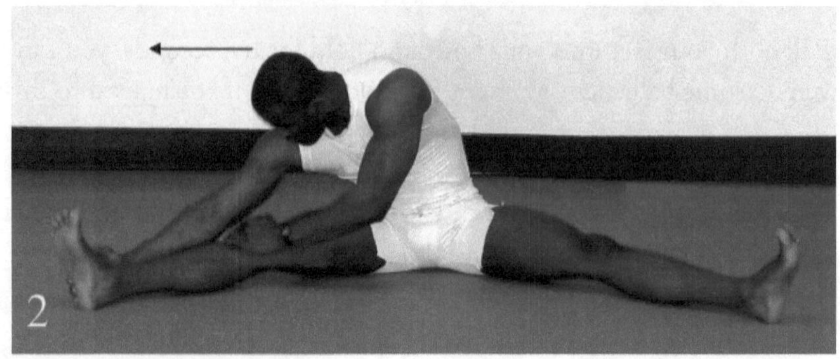

Come up and lean towards your left leg using both hands and grab your foot or ankle. Try to place your chest to your front thigh.

MIDDLE POSITION

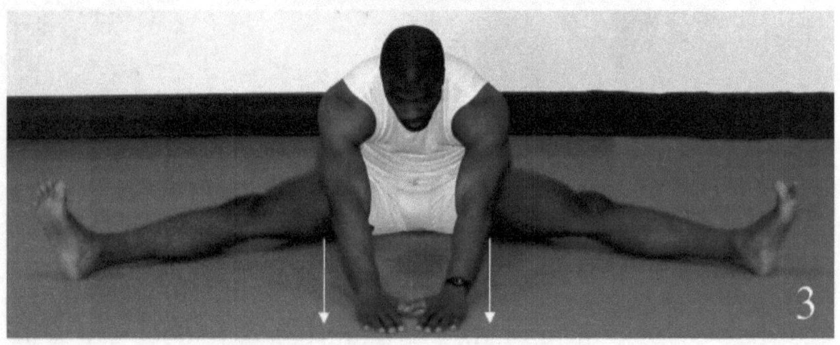

Repeat step 1.

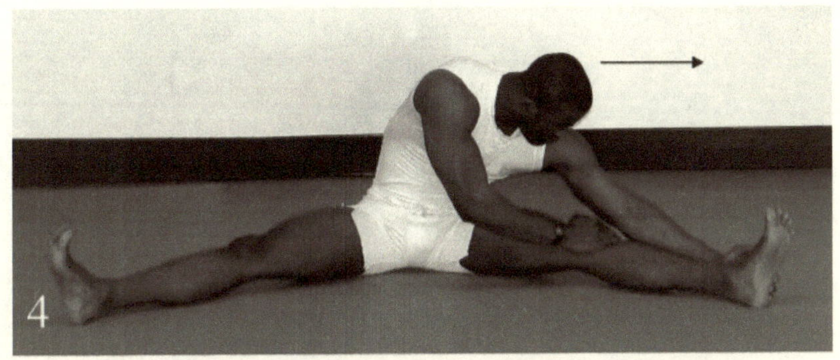

Repeat step 2 but on the opposite side.

Standing Calf Stretching

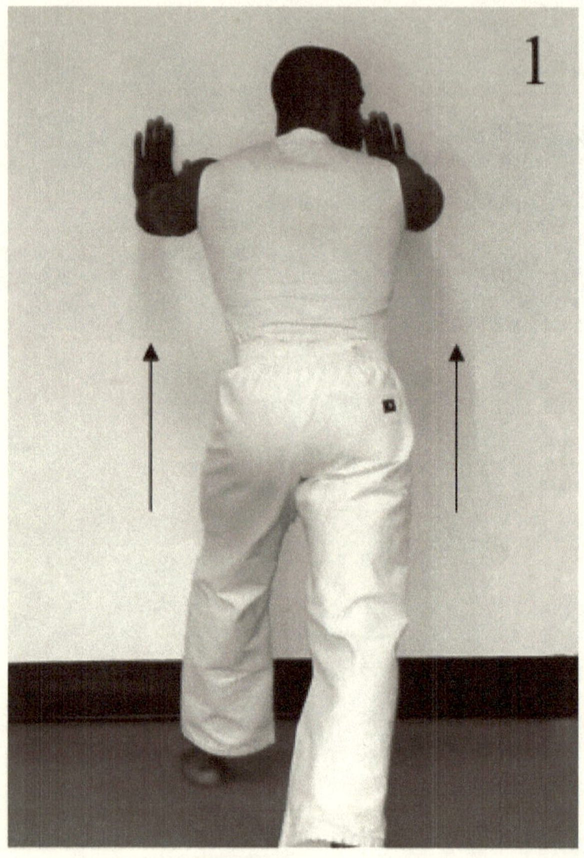

Face the wall in a huge position with both hands against the wall for added support

SIDE VIEW

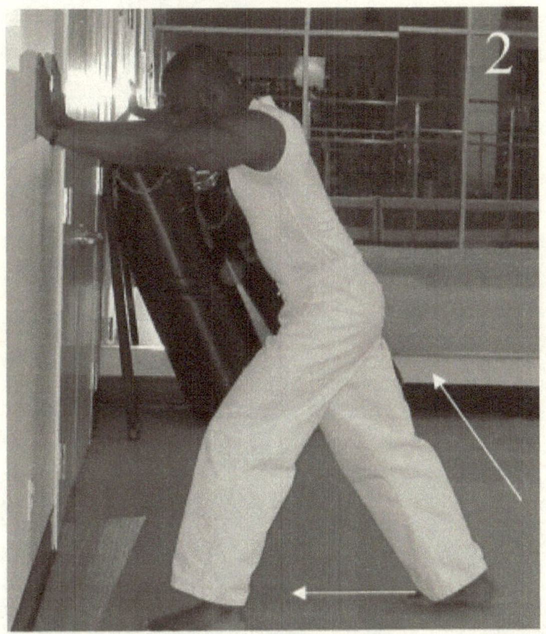

See the side view illustration

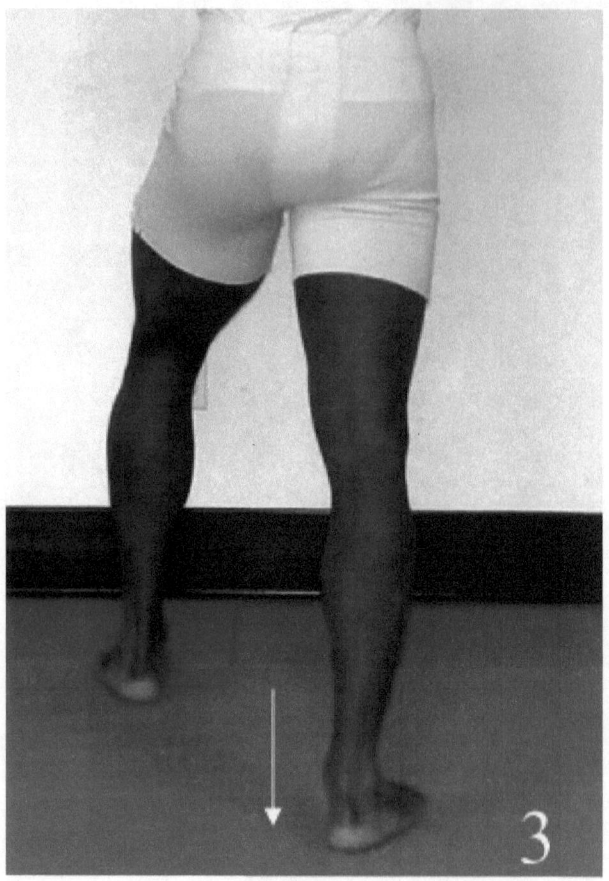

Rise up on the toes of the rear leg and slowly stretch the calf by
lowering your heel.

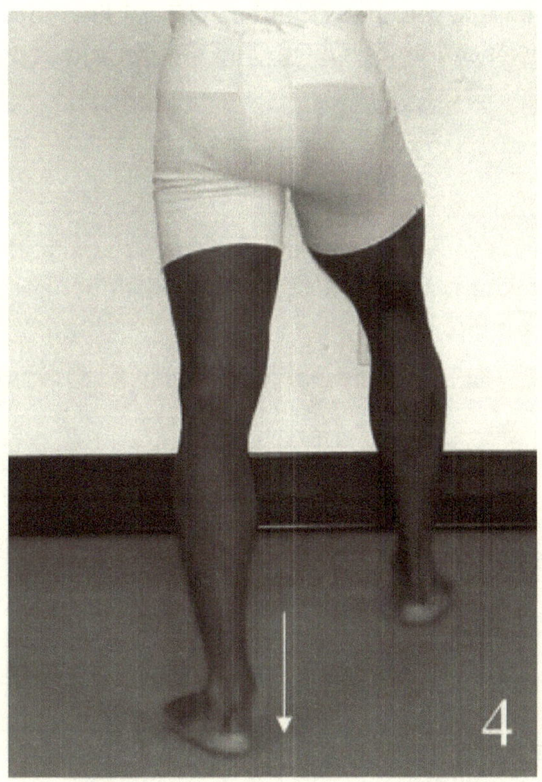

Repeat the same thing on the opposite side.

Note: The further back from the wall you position your back leg, the deeper the calf stretch.

Natural Weight training routines

2.Bodyweight squats

Doing squats will enable you to work the legs and glute muscles. Be careful when doing squats to avoid hurting your knees. Every time you squat, make sure your chest is poked out to make sure your back straight and shoulders are back so you take the strain off your lower back. Also, make sure your butt is pushed out just like when you want to sit in a chair. Then use your thighs and hips muscles to stand up or push yourself up.

Steps

- Stand with your legs apart and the hands placed at the back of your head. Your feet should be slightly apart to open your hip joint.

START & FINISH
POSITION

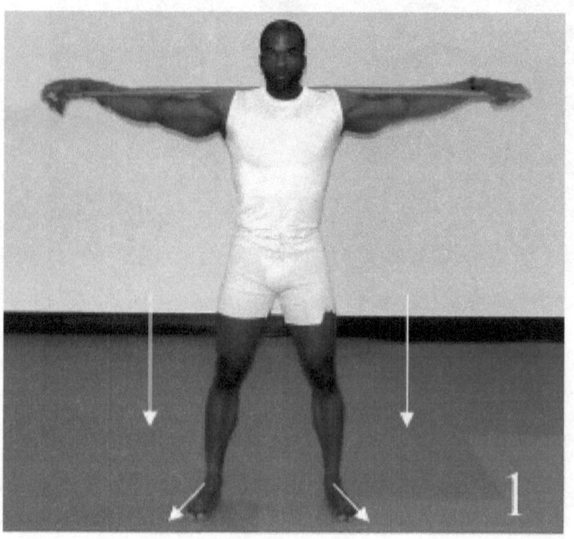

Your feet should be placed slightly past your shoulder line in a parallel stance and the feet at an angle of 15 degrees.

SIDE VIEW

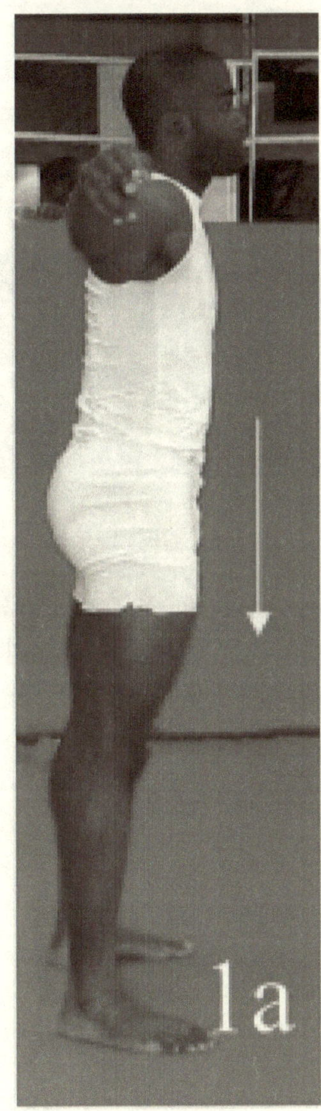

1a. start to release your waist first and then knees in a smooth squatting motion as shown in side view 2a.

MIDDLE POSITION

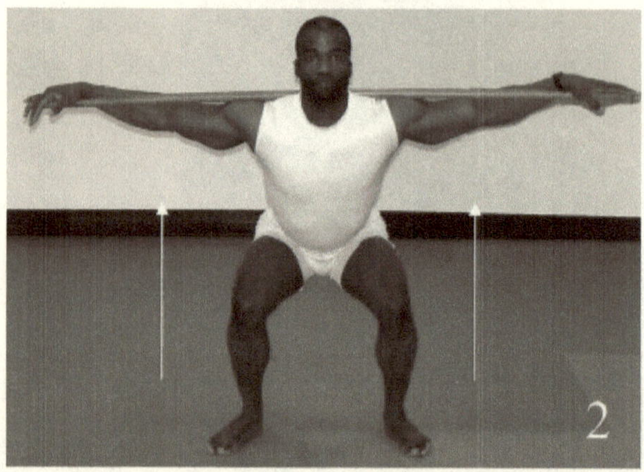

Push back up with both legs equally to return to starting position as shown in diagram 1. When lowering your body, the thighs should be in a 90 degree parallel position to the floor.

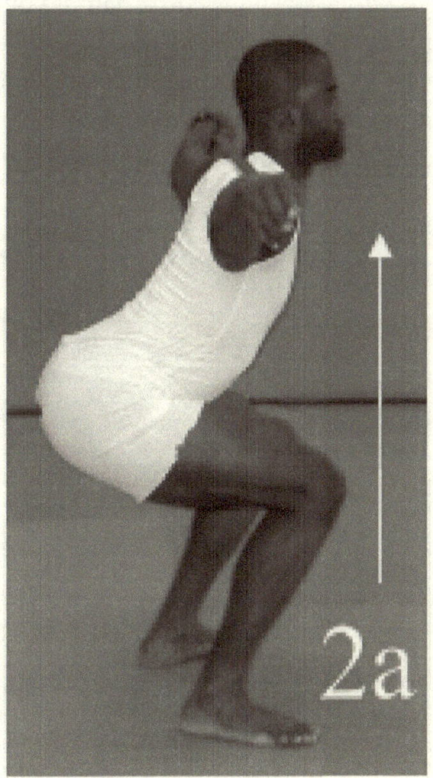

2a. Stay in that position for a few seconds then go back to the starting position. Repeat the process again.

NOTE: My head is up, the chest is pushing out, and my back is not bowed out! When squirting, push up the ward evenly. The position of my knees are the same, they don't move out or collapse at any time. There should be no bouncing during this motion either at the top or bottom of the exercise.

Be careful not to press your knees forward when doing the exercise. Your knees should only move in the first half of your squat, then your hips should support the rest of the movement.

When doing squats, you can challenge yourself by adding plyometric motion like jumps. After squatting to your lowest position, you can jump up allowing you to lift up your both feet off the floor and go back into your starting point.

Squat kicks

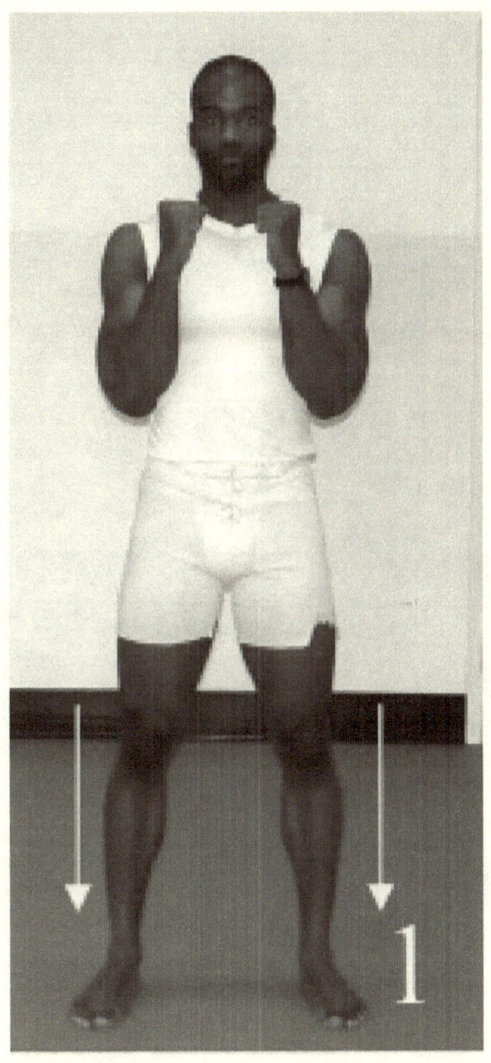

Start by putting your hands up and squatting a regular squat motion.

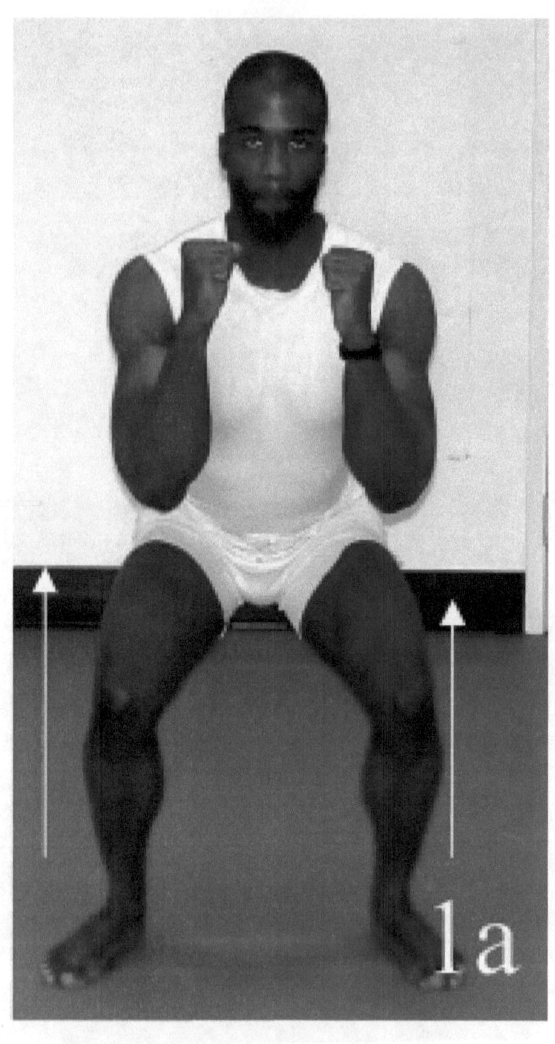

1a. Start moving upward.

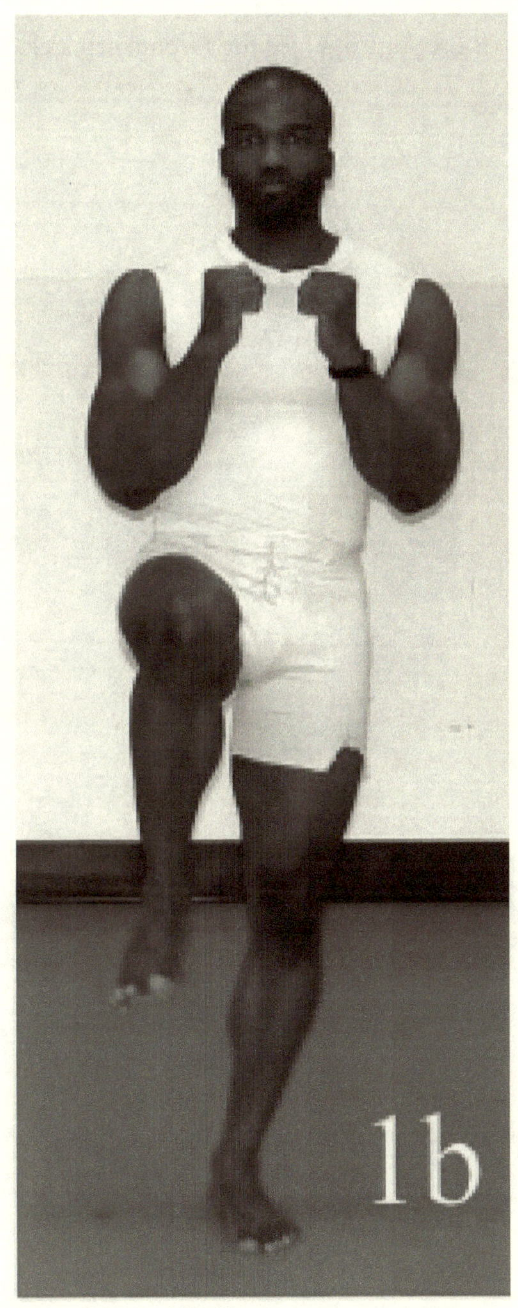
1b

1b. Raise your right leg for a front snap kick.

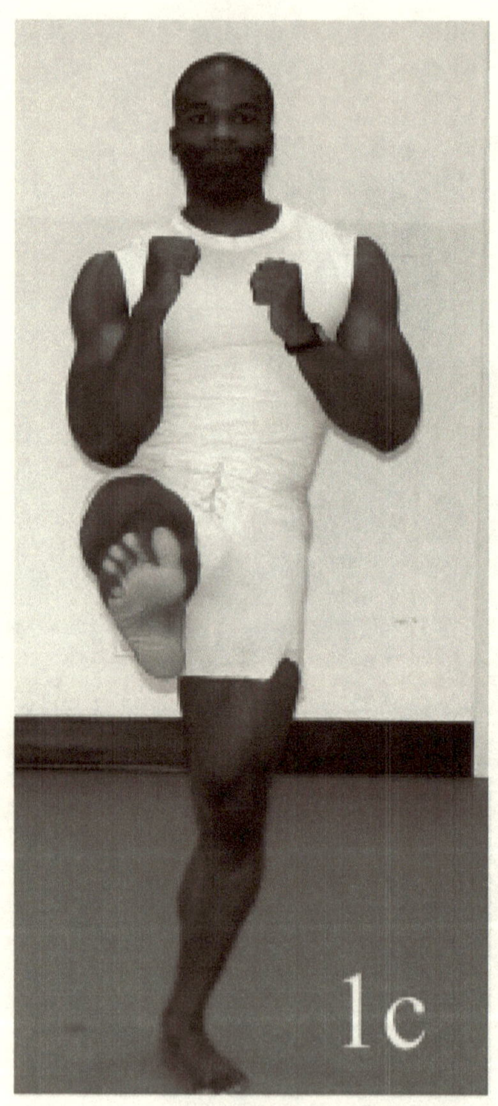

1c. Extend the foot striking with the ball of the foot while holding the position for one second.

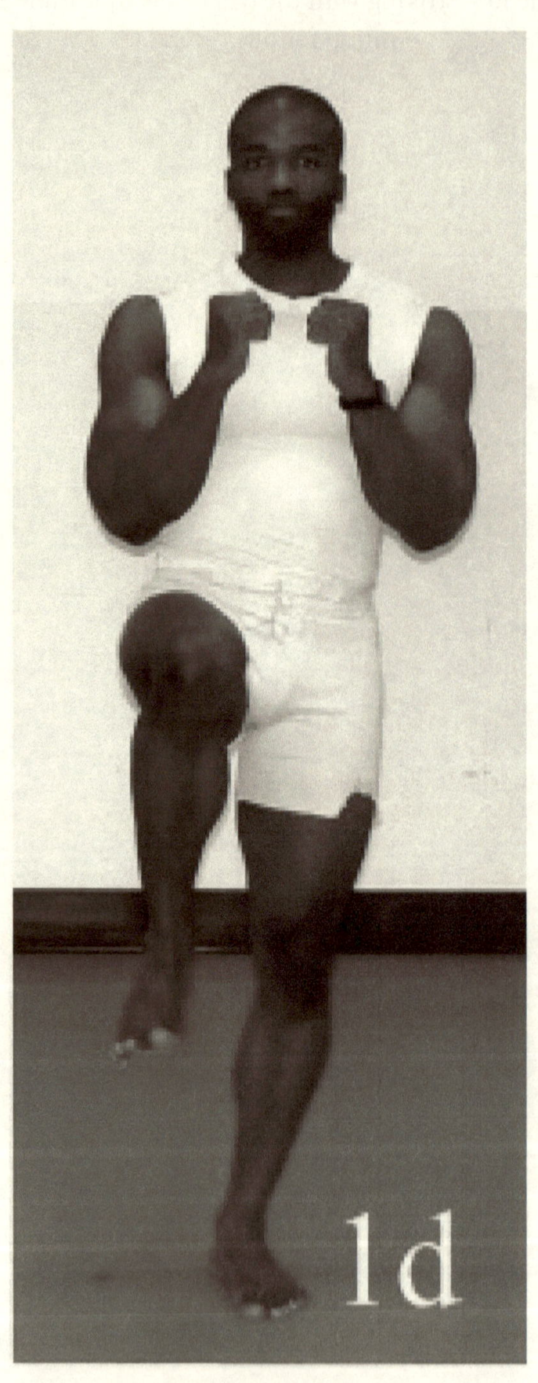
1d

1d. Return the foot back to the position in 1. Get the foot back to the middle position and repeat on the other side.

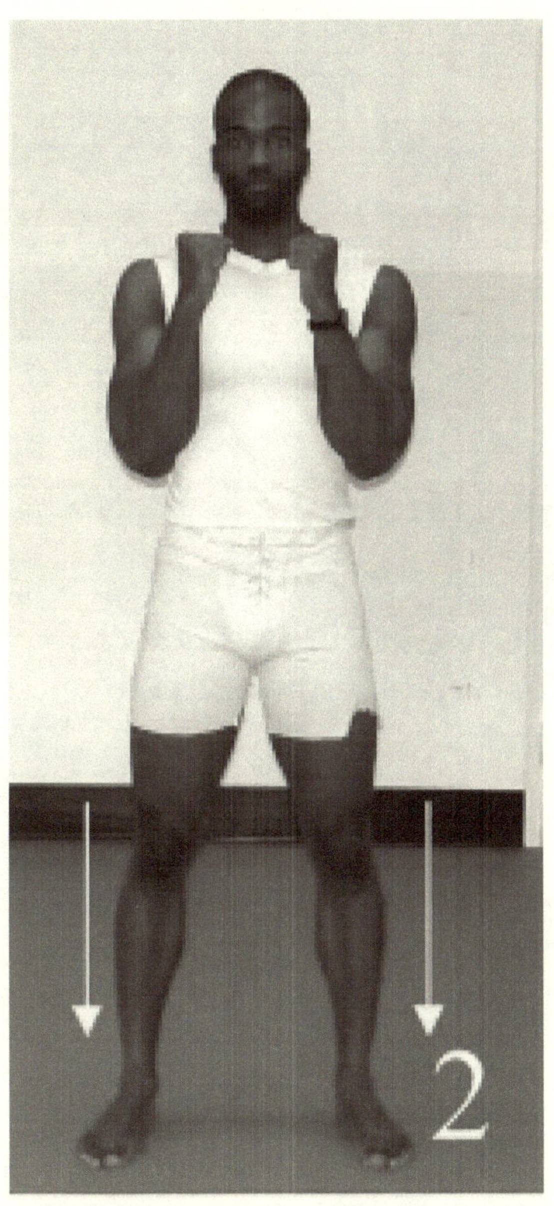

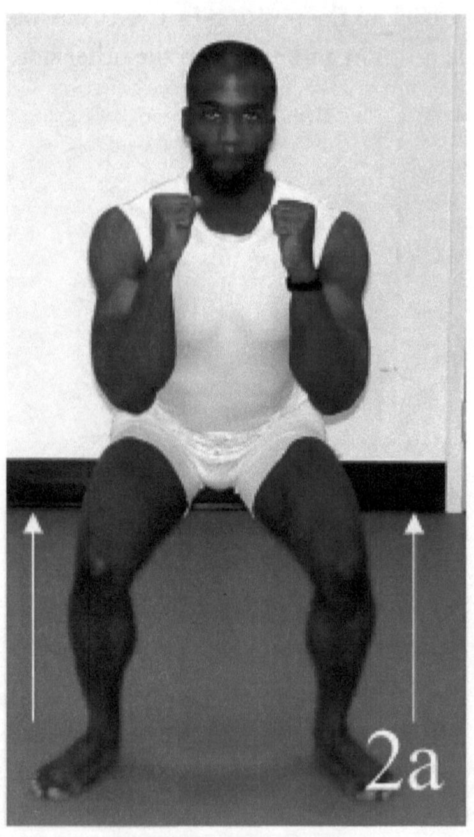

2a

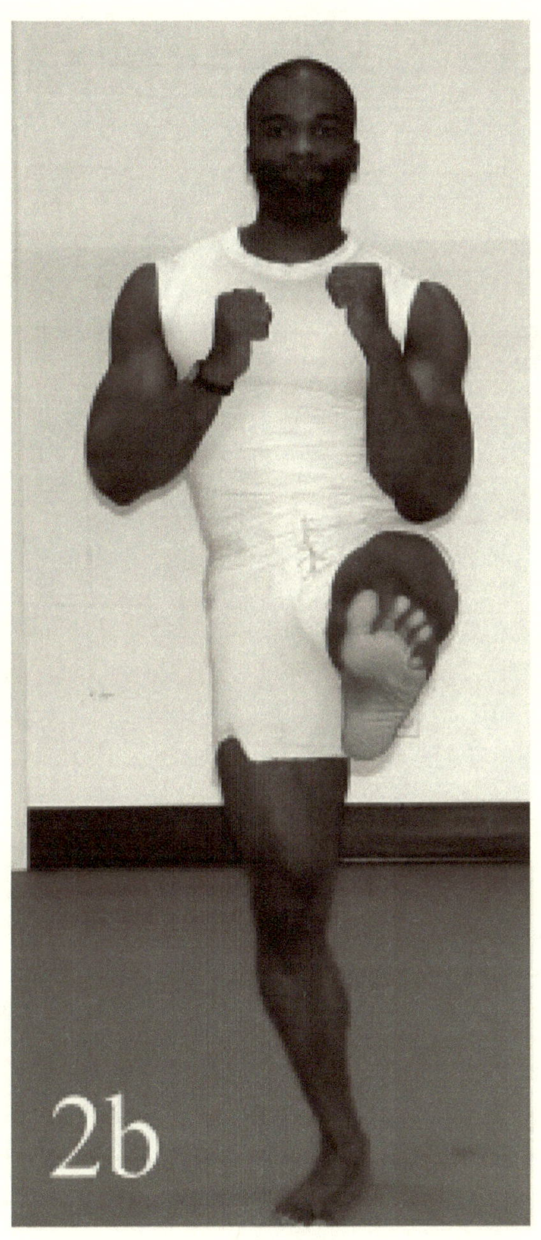

2b

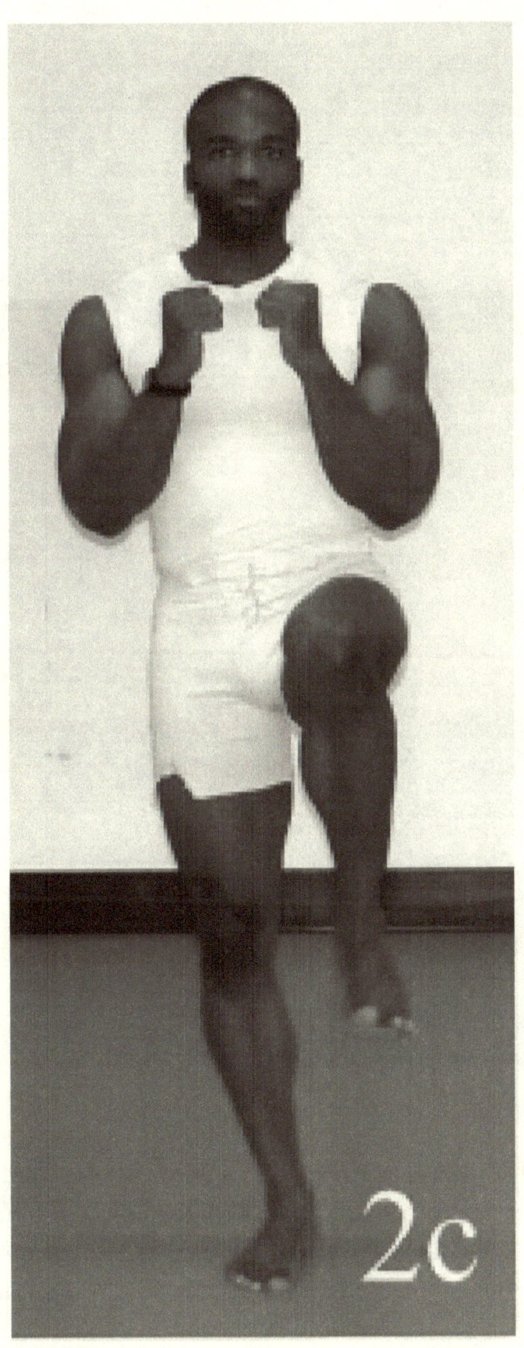

2c

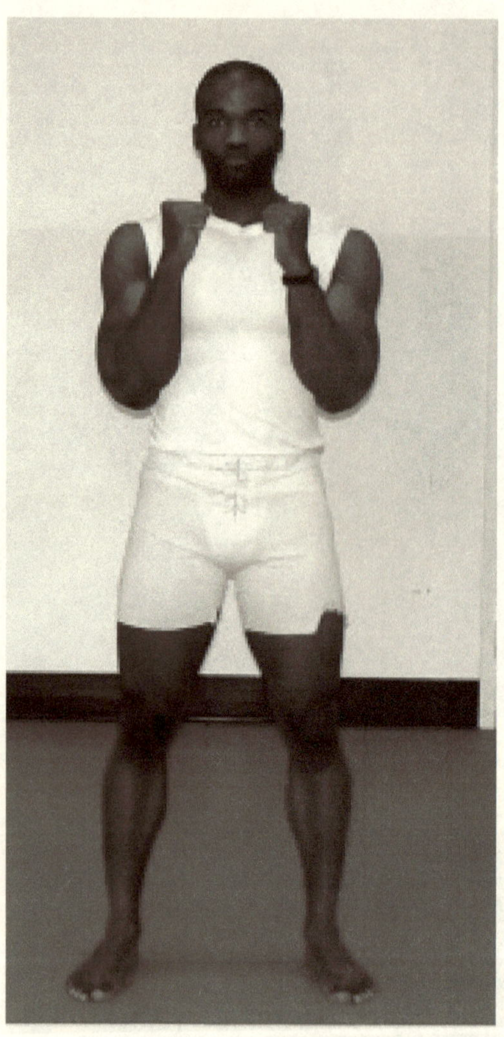

NOTE: The position of my body is upright not leaning in either way. Look at the leg when it is extended. The leg is waist height (if you can extend your leg higher for training purposes that's good, but your maximum energy is at this height); waist level shown on the side view.

SIDE VIEW

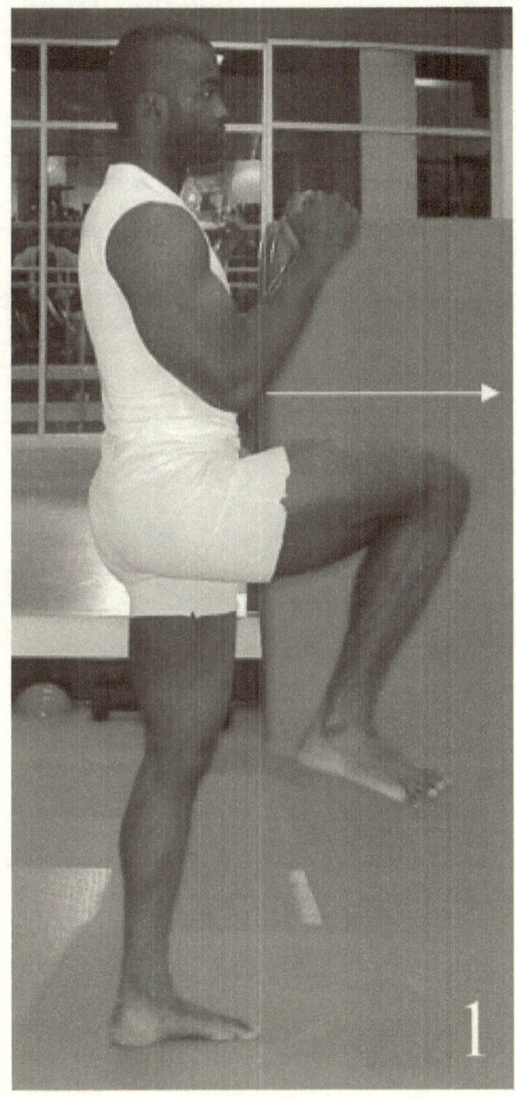

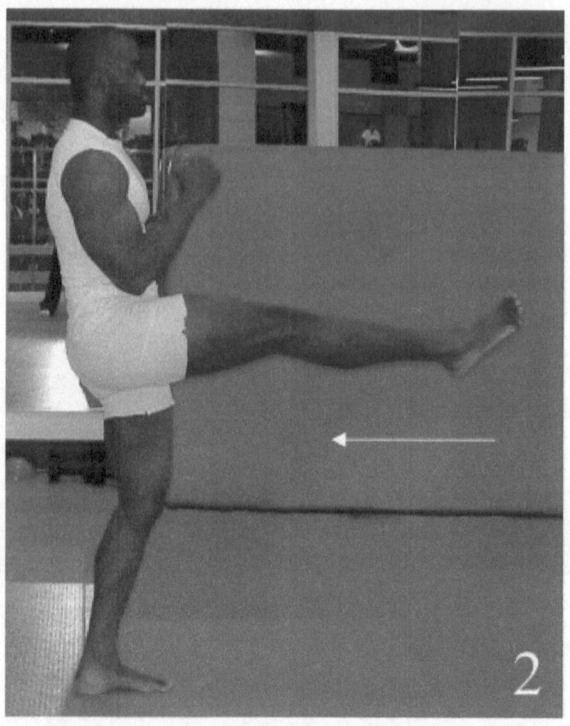

3. Kicks

Side Piercing Kick

START POSITION

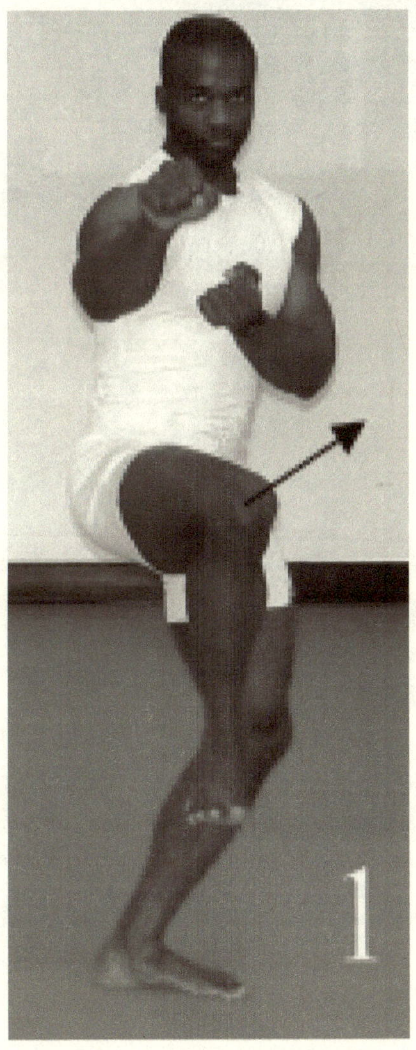

Start in a front-facing guarding stance bringing your left leg up.

SIDE VIEW

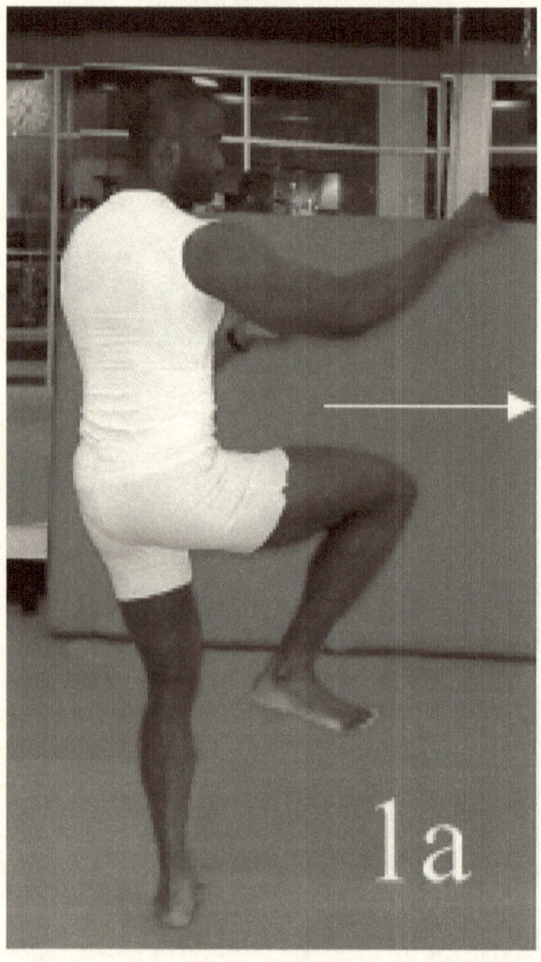

1a. Like in diagram 1. move the knee over so it is horizontal to the floor and push the leg out on a straight motion.

FINISH POSITION

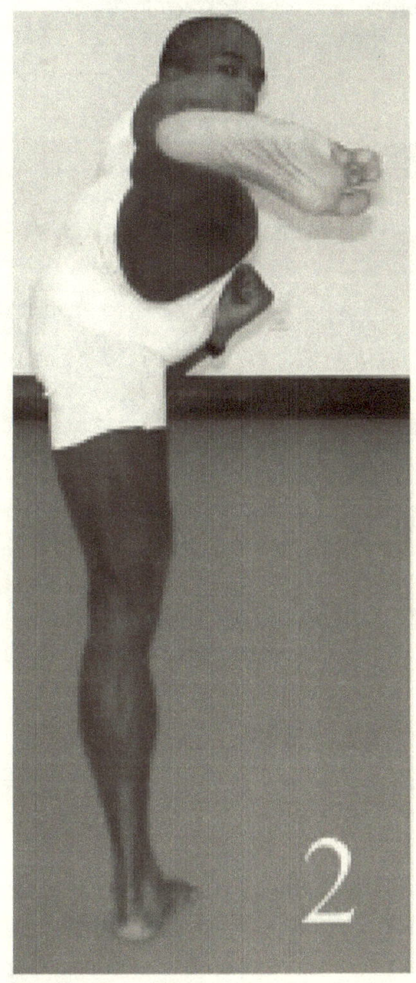

Striking with your heel or foot sword.

SIDE VIEW

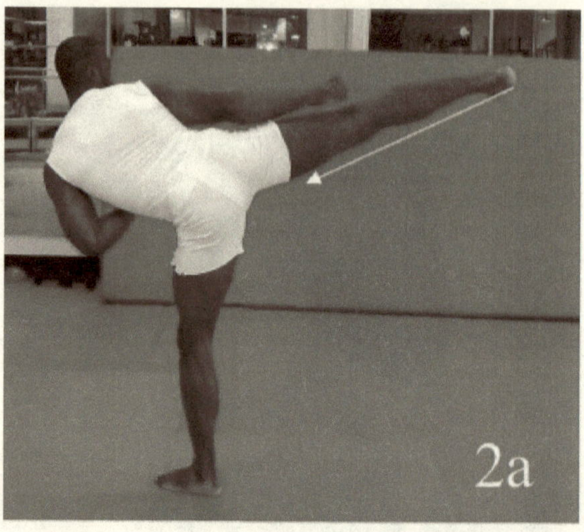

2a. Recoil the leg back to the middle position in 1a. and place the foot back down. This the way to execute a lead or front leg side piercing kick. Pulling or re-chambering the leg where it projected from in diagram 1.

REPEAT the same motion with the opposite leg

NOTE: The position of my body and feet in this motion. If your butt is sticking out too far, then your body is not aligned properly. Also bend your supporting leg before impact and straighten at the point of impact for maximum penetration! Then after the impact, you can bend that leg again for balance.

Side turning or roundhouse kick

START POSITION

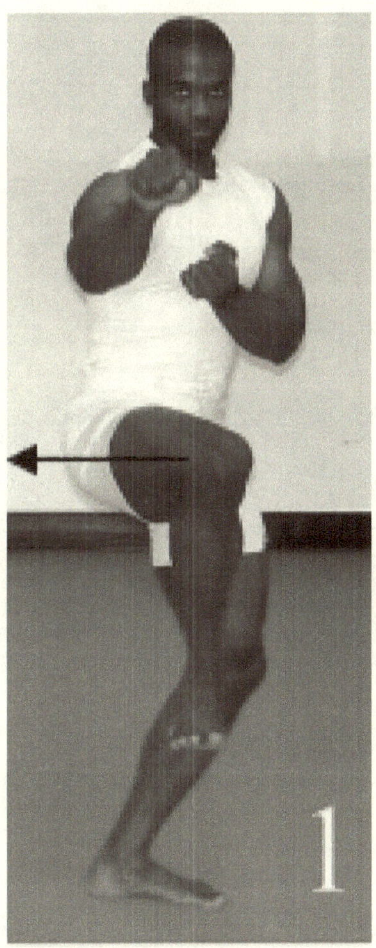

Start in a front-facing guarding stance bringing your left leg up

MIDDLE POSITION

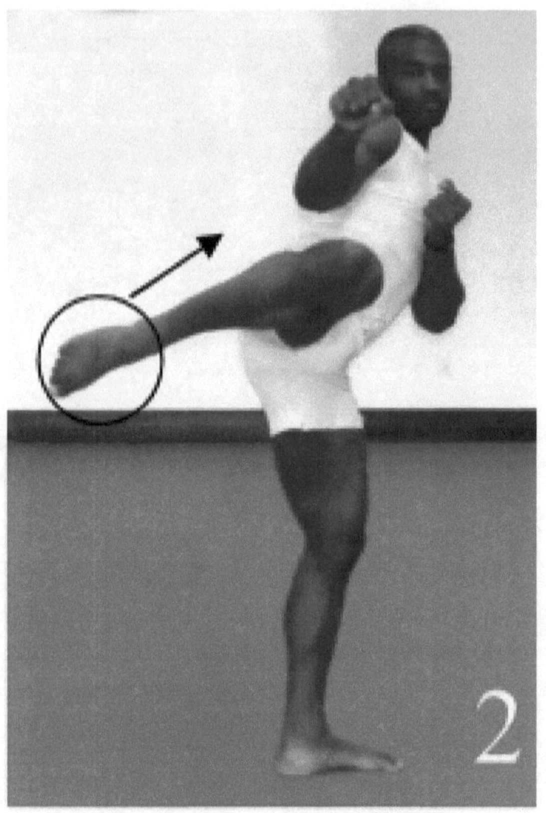

Bring your knee slightly outward first

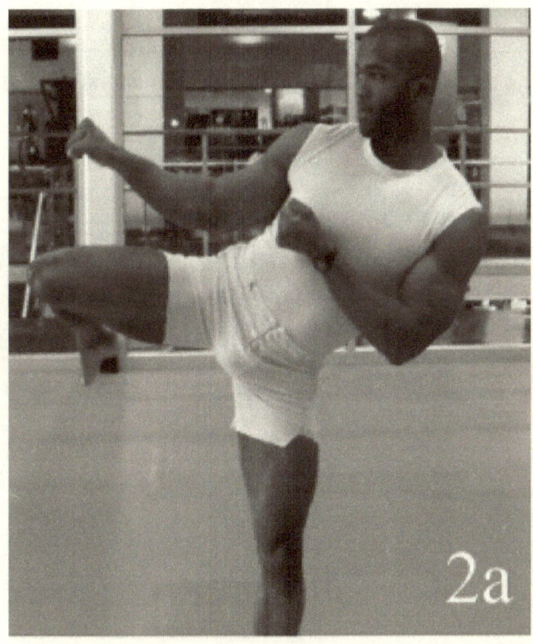

FINISH POSITION

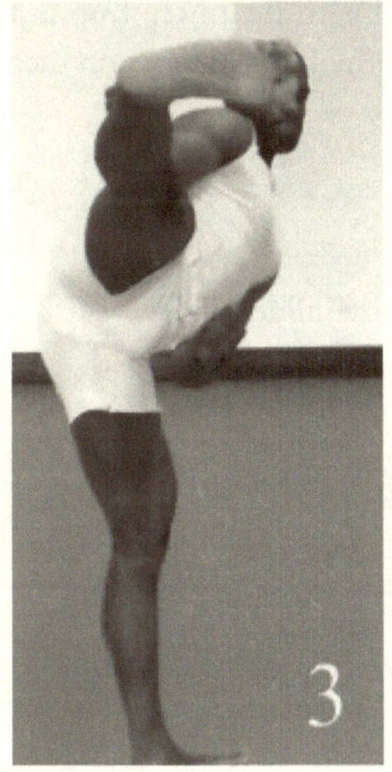

Extend your leg from the motion shown in 2 above as if it were swing or turning to execute the kick. When kicking, strike with the ball of your foot.

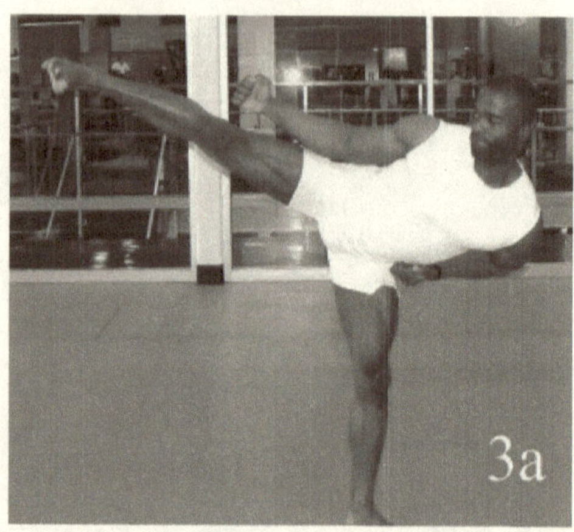

NOTE: Notice the position of my body and feet in this exercise. The striking tool can be performed with the instep (top of the foot) as shown in diagram 2. or the ball of the foot as shown in diagram 3. See the side view on diagram 3a.

4. Push-ups/ press-ups

Push-ups are very great for bodybuilders. They help you work on your chest and shoulder muscles.

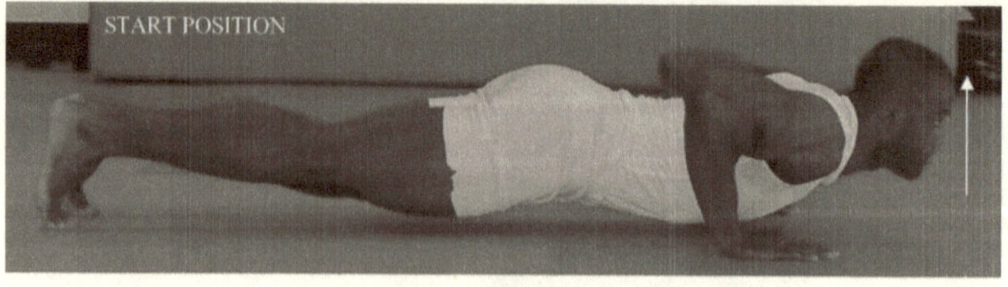

Steps

- Get down on all fours
- Extend your hands to be in an equal distance apart but not too far and directly underneath the shoulders, not over the shoulders and not too far under. Try and make a direct line with your palms slightly under your shoulders so you don't strain your wrist or elbows while performing this motion.
- Stretch your legs and arms to be straight
- Lower your body until you're almost touching the floor with your chest.
- Hold in that position for a second and push yourself up to the starting point.
- Repeat the process with as many reps as desired.

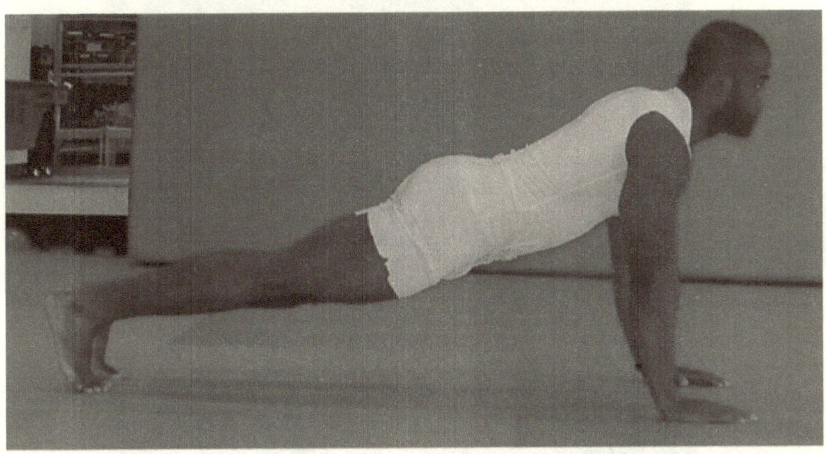

NOTE: The position of my hands are slightly under or in a straight line to my shoulders. Also, my body doesn't rest on the ground, it stays slightly alleviated and my chin is up with my back tensed never moving down or bowing upwards.

If you find it difficult to do the standard push-ups, you can put your knees on the floor and try again. This will help you reduce the amount of weight you have to lift.

When doing the push-ups you can also squeeze your abs and glutes muscle. This will build your core and increase more tension in your body maximizing your efficiency in building muscle mass and strength.

For a more challenging exercise, you can place your feet on a block and increase the intensity of the exercise.

5. Back & Biceps Workout

Pull-ups

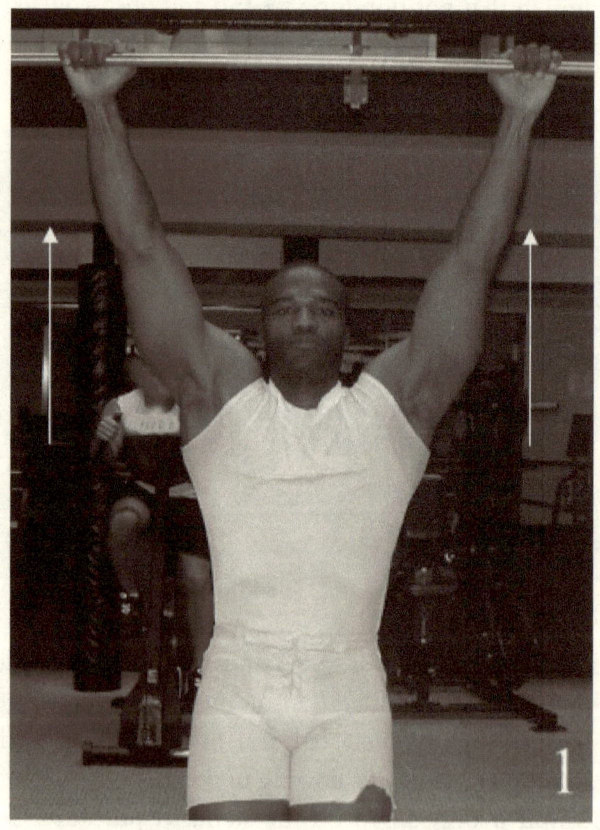

Make sure your hands are even with the bar and pull upwards.

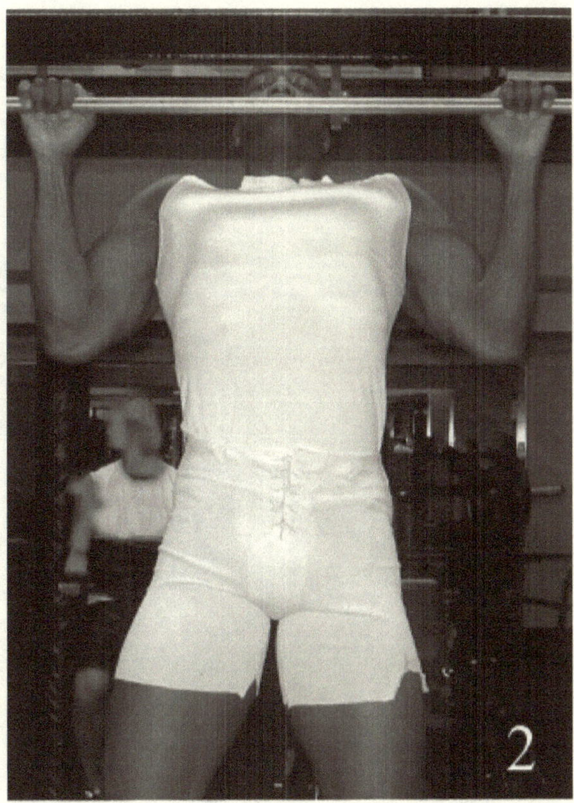

Pause for a second and repeat the motion from 1 to 2 for as men reps
as you desire.

NOTE: The motion should be smooth and the body should NOT
be swinging! By changing your hands' position and switching the grip,
and having your palms face you is called "CHIN UP". This allows you
to work your Biceps during that exercise. Keep the movement smooth
and natural. Push or poke your chest out on every movement to target
your lats.

6. Calves & Abs

Calves raise

START POSITION

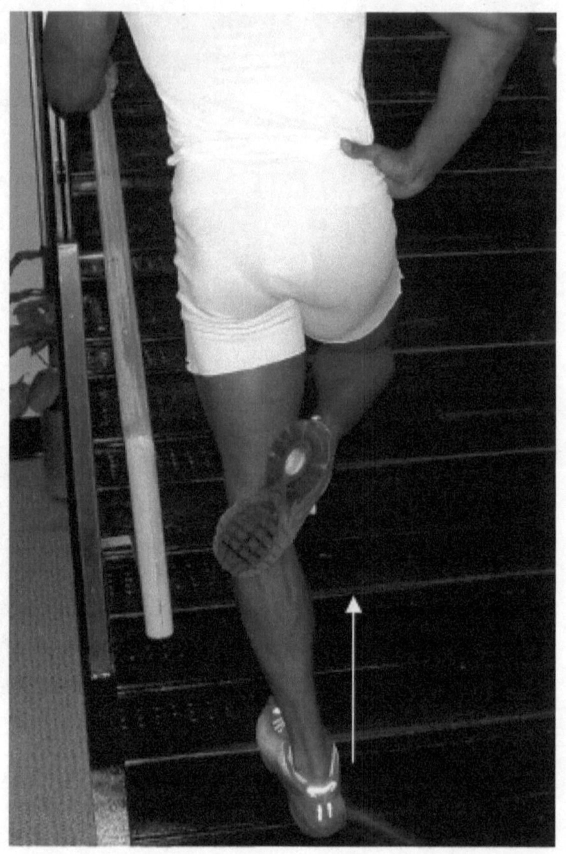

Place one hand on your waist and the other on a handrail. Put your foot behind your knee and the edge of your foot on a step or elevated ledge and raise the working foot upwards.

FINISH POSITION

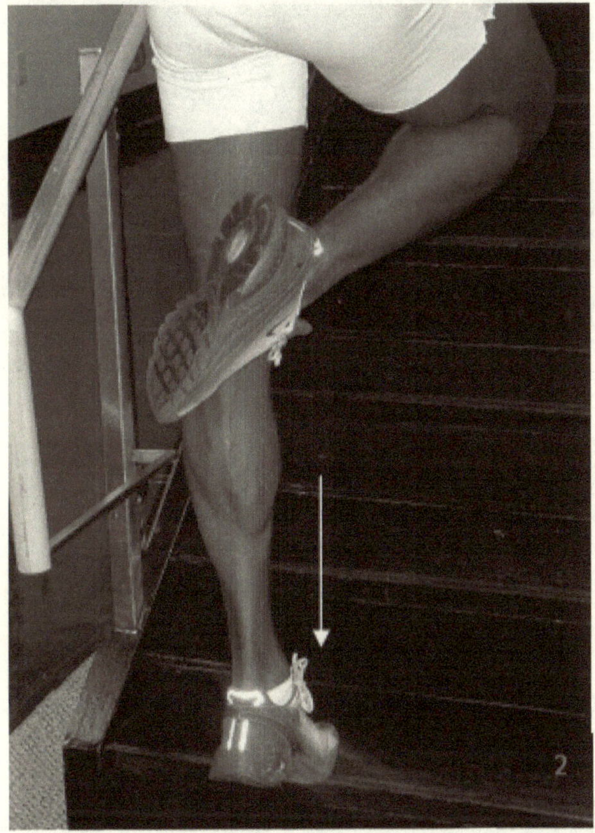

Lower and repeat for 5 reps. Switch and then do with the other leg.

Abs & Lower Back

START POSITION

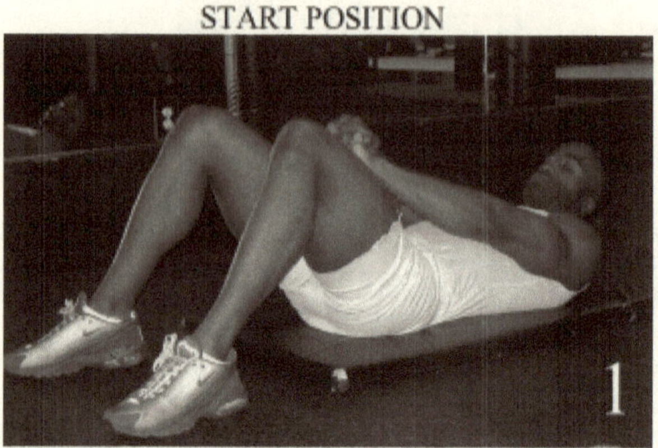

Start on your back in an Ab crunch position with both feet on the floor and your hand interlocked (both palms facing down).

FINISH POSITION

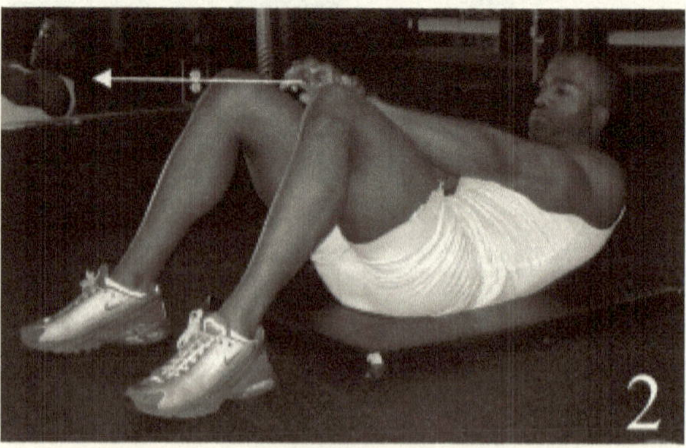

Contract your abs by pushing your hands through your legs and bringing your shoulders slightly off the ground. Then repeat the motion.

NOTE: If your lower back comes off the ground, then you have gone up too far!

Side Midsection, oblique & lower back

START POSITION

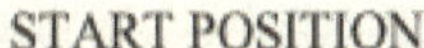

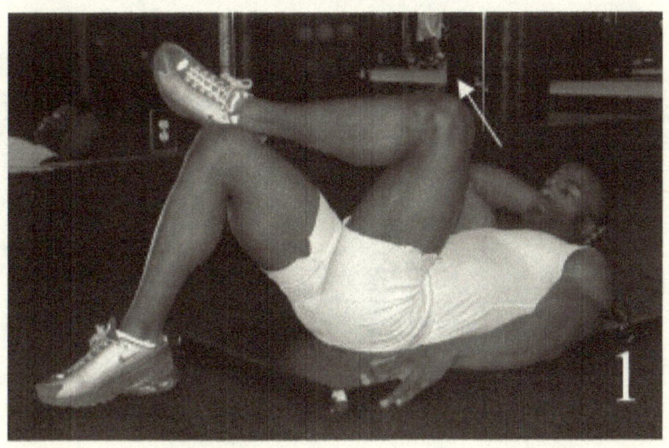

Place your left foot on your right knee.

FINISH POSITION

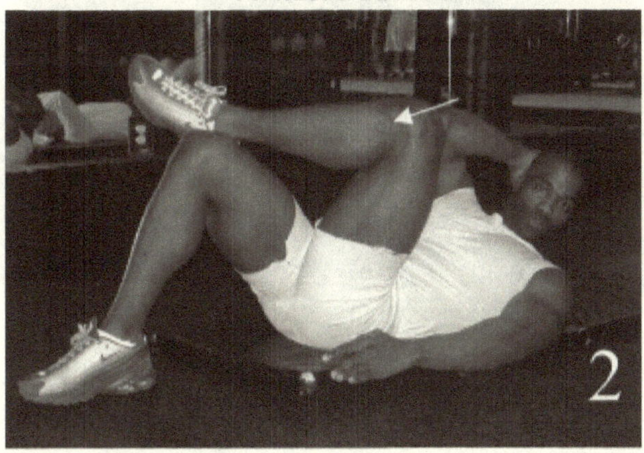

Bring your right elbow to your left knee.

REPEAT on the other side for as many reps as desired.

Stretching your lower back

START POSITION

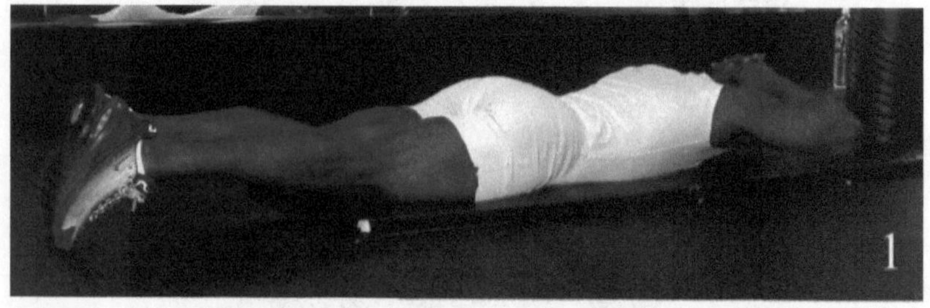

Lay on your stomach interlocking your fingers behind your head or neck.

FINISH POSITION

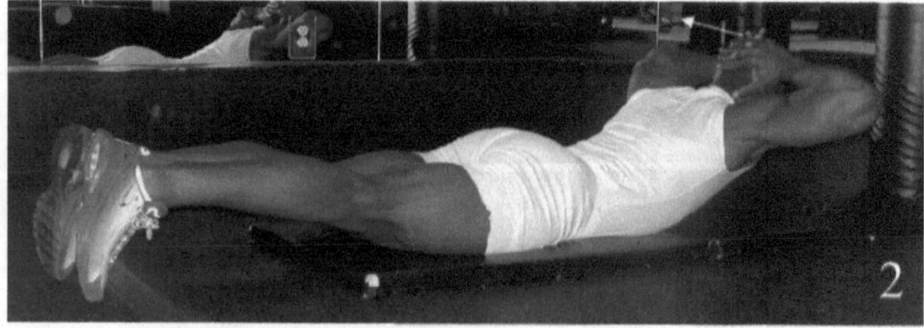

Raise your chest off the ground as far you can go comfortably and return to the start position.

Note: There should be no swinging movement, move naturally.

7. Forward Toe Touch

START POSITION

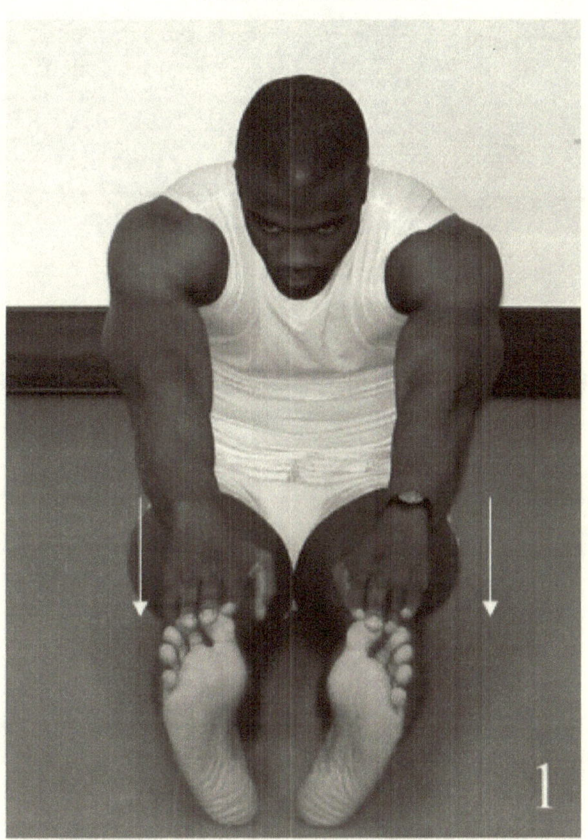

Just like in gym class when you were a little kid, the goal is to lean forward as far as you can go and touch your toes or grab your feet.

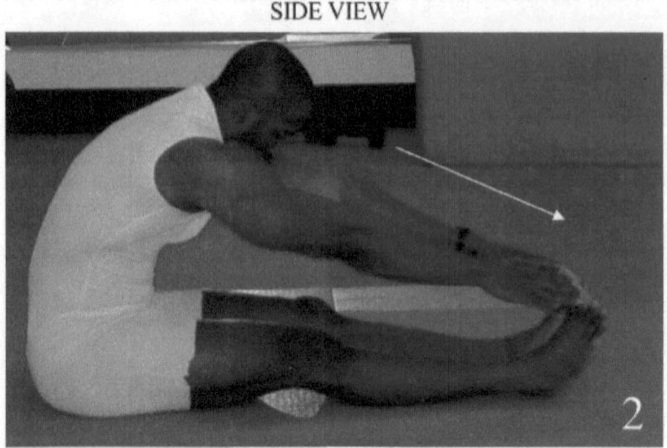

By trying to touch your chest to your thighs or knees will maximize your stretch position.

8. Leg raises

Leg raise exercises allow you to reduce your back pains as it gives an opportunity to press your lower back on the floor while working on your abs. In this form of exercise, your core will do most of the work instead of the hips thus reducing any back pain. To obtain desired results from this form of exercise, your legs should move in a controlled manner throughout the entire exercise.

Steps

Lie on your back with your legs together and straight

START POSITION

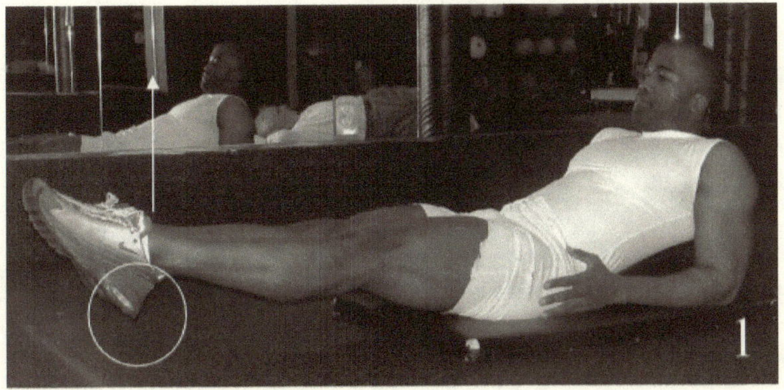

Start by sitting up on your elbows and placing your hands next to your waist. If you have a martial arts uniform on, grab your belt with both hands from the side. Elevate your feet six inches off the floor.

MIDDLE POSITION

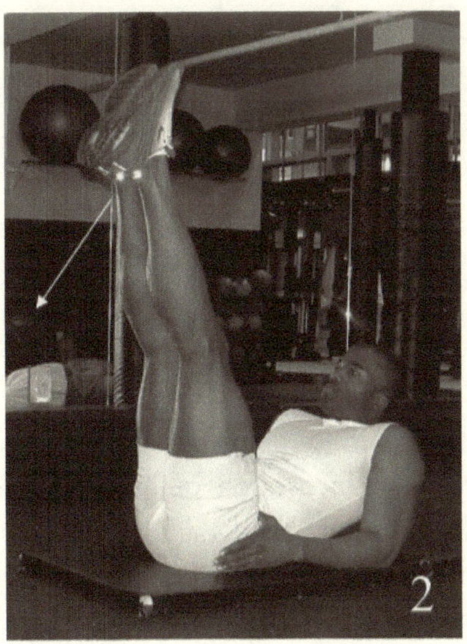

Keep your legs straight and feet 6 inch off the floor. The feet should be raised at 90 degrees from the floor.

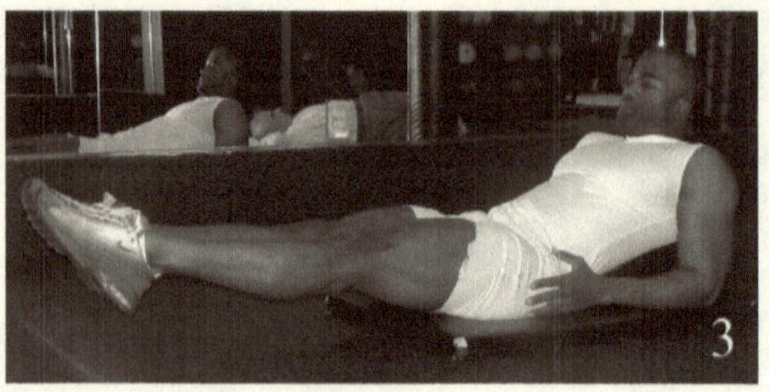

Lower your feet back to the start position as shown in figure 1. (Lower the legs down until they are slightly above the floor and hold on for a while). Do NOT rest them on the floor. Keep them 6 inches off the floor.

RAISE your legs back up again and repeat the process

Set 2 Workouts

Take a 1-minute break and continue with this set of exercises.

1. Plank

The plank exercise helps you tone your abs and build your upper body strength. It focuses on building your shoulders, arms, and legs muscles. In addition, planks allow you to simultaneously strengthen abdominal and low back muscles.

Planks are highly recommended for people suffering from low back pains.

Planks can be more effective when done on your forearm because they can cause some harm to your wrist.

You can make the planks more comfortable by placing your knees on the floor in order to reduce the amount of weight being put on your forearms.

Steps

- Lie down on a flat surface with your front.
- Raise your body to assume a push-up position then bend your arms on the elbow to allow your weight rest on your forearms.
- Clench your glute muscles and tighten your abs to train your core.
- Ensure your body is kept straight from head to your feet.
- Hold on in the position for a minute or as long as you can.
- Lower yourself down and take a breath.

2. Lunges or Jump Lunges

This is another form of squat that supports the quadriceps and hamstring muscles found on your legs and glutes. Adding jumps from your lowest point into the starting position when squatting will lead to a plyometric boost.

Steps

- Place your both hands on your hips.
- Take a step forward with the left leg to provide you with enough balance.
- Slowly lower your body and lower as you can
- After getting to your lowest point, jump up with enough force to lift both feet off the floor.
- Then land with your right leg forward.
- Alternate your legs and repeat the steps.

If you find it hard to balance yourself during the exercise, you can move close to a wall to allow your hands to rest on the wall for support.

If you find this type of exercise hard on your knees, you can do away with a plyometric jump. But if you can successfully include jumps without any problem, you can challenge yourself by jumping higher. As a result, you will boost your cardio intensity as well as boost your strength.

3. Single leg hip raise

A single-leg hip raise targets your glute muscles and abs. When doing this type of exercise, ensure the other foot is firmly placed on the floor.

Steps:

- Lie on a flat surface with your back and bend your right knee and place it flat on the floor.
- Raise up the left leg and ensure it is in-line with the right thigh.
- Push your hips up and ensure the left leg remains elevated.
- Stay in that position for 10 seconds then slowly go back to the starting position
- Switch the legs and repeat the exercise again

You can challenge yourself by placing your foot on a bench or step to enable you to raise your hips higher.

Set 3:

After doing the second set of exercises, you can take a minute break and continue with the last set of exercises.

1. Burpee with push-ups

Burpee exercises are great for your entire body and will get your heart pumping faster. This form of exercise is more effective when done in slow motion. Doing it too quickly will leave you gasping for breath. Just go with moderate speed and have complete control of your body as you continue with the exercises.

Burpee is a great exercise for burning calories due to a lot of energy required to do the exercise.

Steps

- Stand with your feet at shoulder-width apart
- Lower your body to a squatting position and place the hands on the floor.
- Stretch your legs out behind you until you're in a push-up position and do a single push-up
- Return your legs back to the squatting position and jump up at the same time through your hands above your head.
- Repeat the steps 5 more times.

After succeeding in this form of workout, you can include 3 o'clock 9 o'clock leg modification. In this case, you can place your right leg into the 3 o'clock position and then return it to the center position, then place the left leg into the 9 o'clock position and then bring it back to the center and do push-ups.

You can do these much faster by stretching your legs back before the hands reach the ground. You shouldn't arch your back when doing the squats to give full range motion to your legs.

2. Single leg-toe touch

This type of exercise allows you to tone your lower body. It helps you target your hamstrings as well as improve your balance.

Steps

- Stand with your right leg while the left leg should be slightly behind you and raised off the floor.
- Stretch your arms straight on your sides and at shoulder height.

- Bend the knee of your right leg and then squat down so that you're able to touch the toe with your left hand. Try as much to keep your left leg raised off the floor and behind you.
- Repeat the step again with your left leg.

You can also do the exercise next to a wall to provide you with enough support you need.

NOTE: As with this movement or any other exercise if you feel pain while training and workout out stop! You must be doing something wrong or your body is out of alignment, causing the pain. You should always be slightly uncomfortable (meaning, from fatigue for muscle burn) when training but never in real pain.

3. Mountain climbing

This type of workout mimics motions made by climbers as they climb a steep mountain peak. In this case, the motions are done on a flat and soft surface on the floor. Mountain climbing exercises provide you with a full-body workout. It allows you to work on your back, arms, and legs muscles, strengthen your core and your heart.

- Place both your hands and knees on the floor
- Put the right foot close to your right hand and slightly stretch your left leg behind you.
- In one swift motion, switch the legs while keeping the hands in the same position.
- Keep shifting your legs back and forth two more times, such that the right leg is always close to the right hand.

When doing this workout, it can put a lot of strain on your wrists. This can be avoided by placing your hands on a step to elevate your upper body and reduce the amount of weight placed on your arms.

Weight Lifting & Resistance Training Routines

Chest, Shoulders & Triceps

Chest (Bench Press)

START POSITION

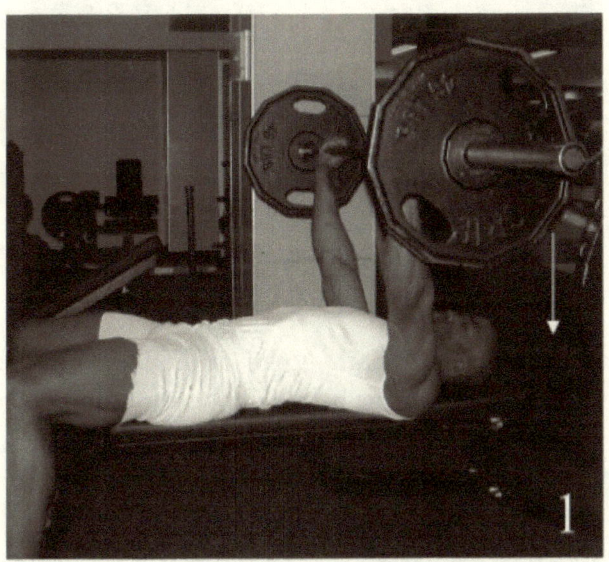

Start by making sure your hands are measured evenly on the barbell and lift the weight off the rack. Make sure you balance properly with your feet flat on the floor.

Note: My back is straight at all times. It should never move up or down. If this happens, then lower the weight!

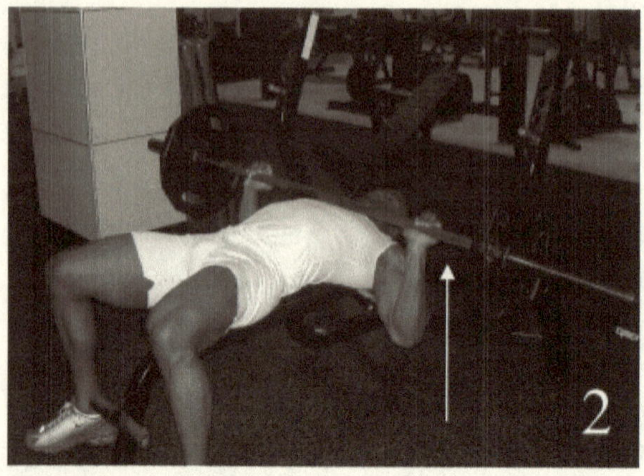

Lower the weight in a smooth motion to the chest. Inhale as the weight is being lowered. The bar should be lowered to the middle section of your chest not low towards the stomach and not too high towards your neck.

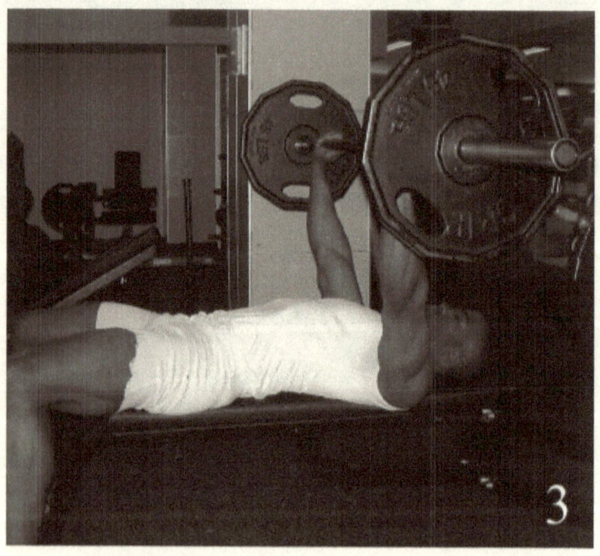

Push the weight and exhale as you move the weight upward. Repeat this motion for as many reps and sets as desired.

Note: There should be no bouncing or jerking of the weight. The weight should never be bounced off your chest at any time during this exercise.

Chest (Dumbbell Flyes)

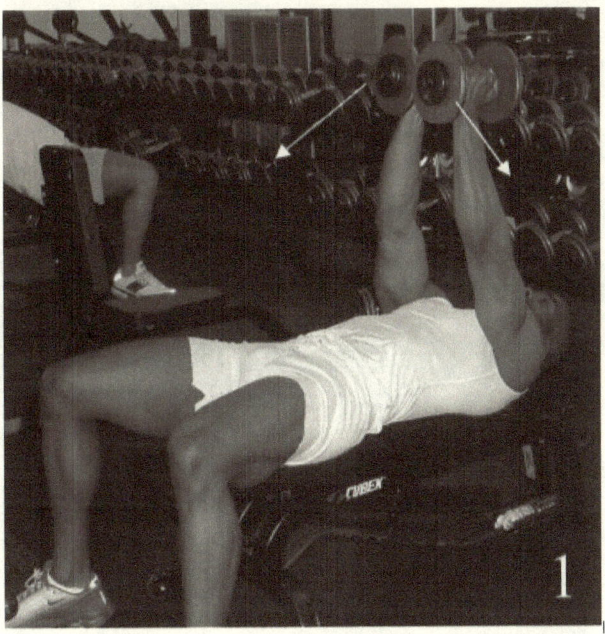

Start this exercise by raising the dumbbells above your chest. Make sure you are using a weight that you can move in both motions.

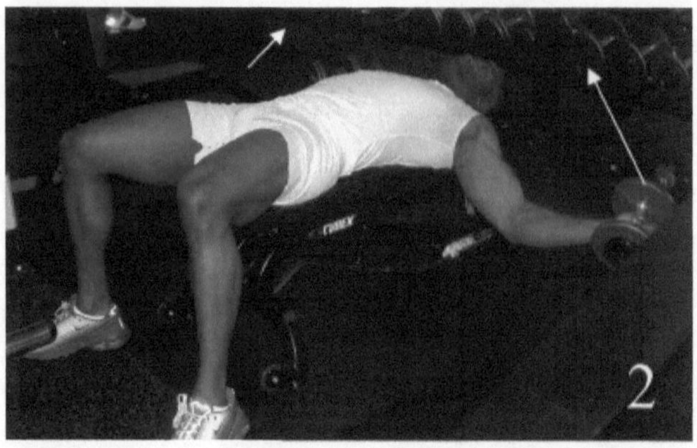

Slowly lower the weight to the point of full pectoral stretch. Inhale as the weight is moving downward.

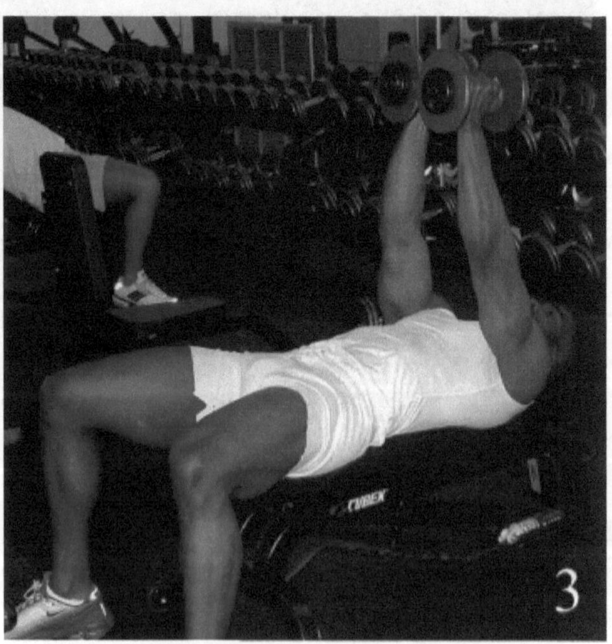

Exhale as the weight is being moved upward and contract the chest muscle in the return position for a half of a second. Repeat the motion as many times as desired for reps and sets.

Note: This is a very dangerous exercise if not done properly due to the fact the weight can put a lot of stress and strain on the shoulder and joints. Keep your arm slightly bent at all times. Control the weight, don't ever let the weight control you!

Shoulders (Barbell Shoulder or Military Press)

START POSITION

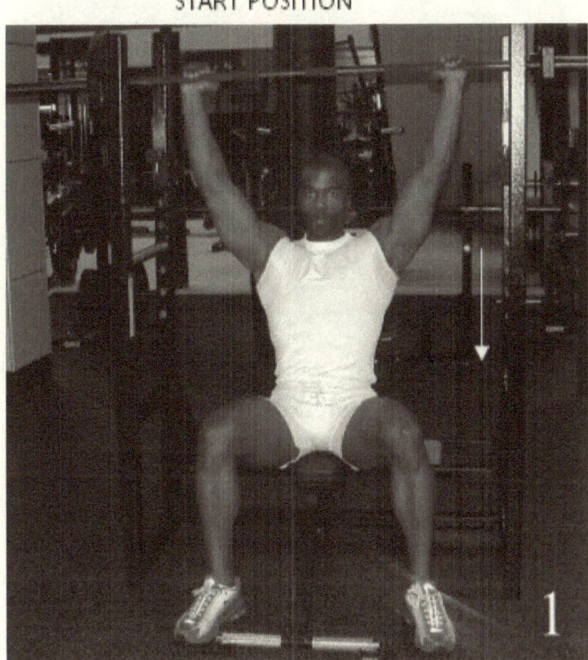

Make sure your hands are even on the barbell and lift the weight off the rack. As you lower the weight inhale. The barbell should be almost touching your shoulders. See Diagram 2.

MIDDLE POSITION

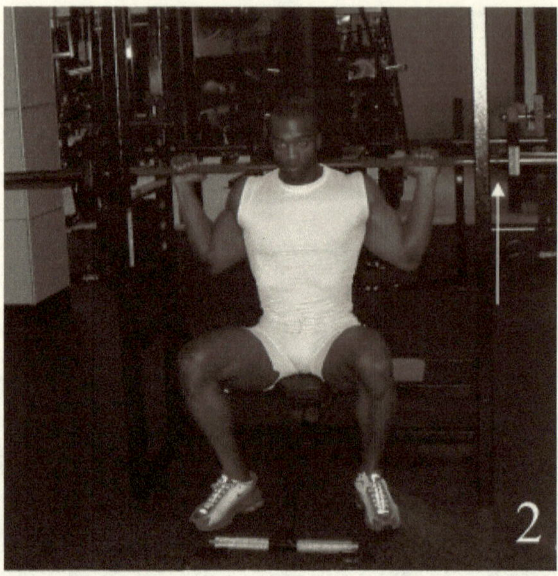

As you push the weight upward, you should be exhaling snd controlling the movement.

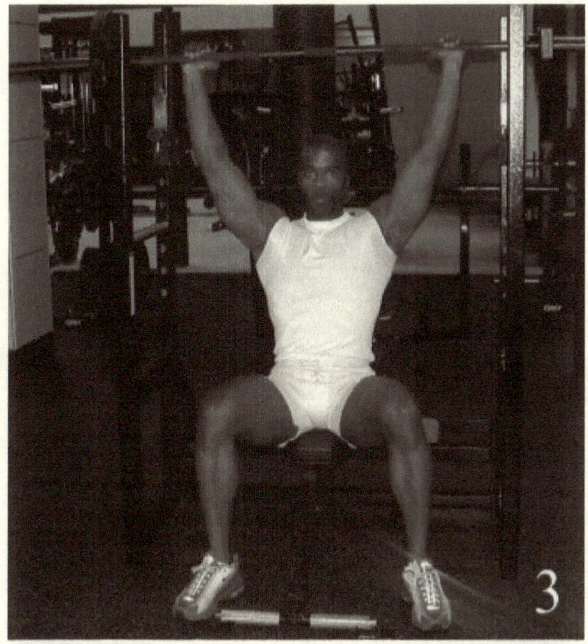

Note: Make sure your back is straight and your feet are in a solid base position not moving as you are moving the weight. The weight should never be lowered without complete control or the barbell. It could hit and hurt your neck and trapezoids as it is lowered in that area recklessly!

Shoulders (Dumbbell Side Lateral Raises)

START POSITION

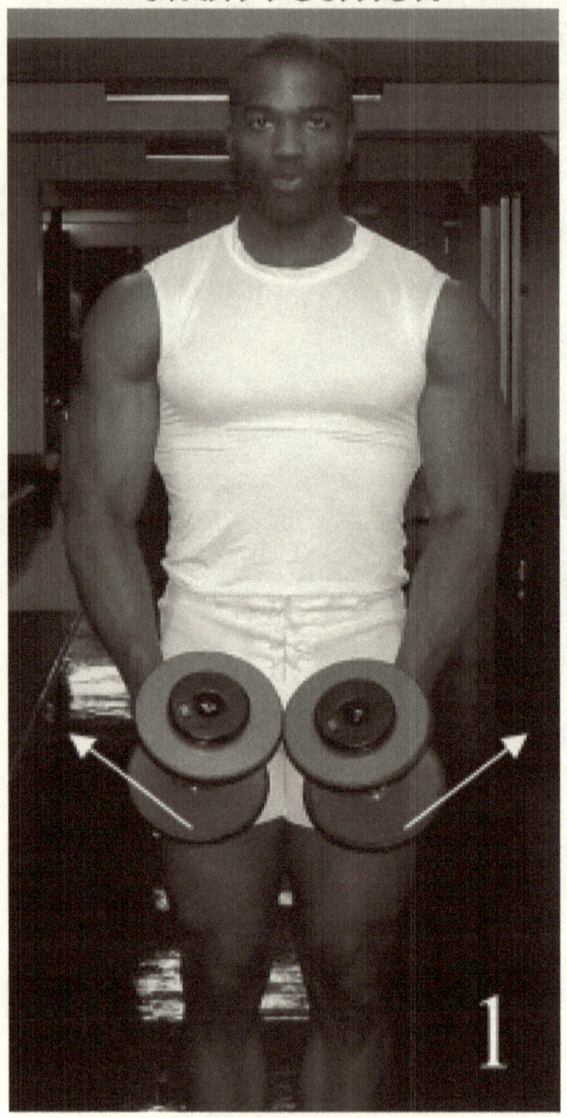

Start by holding the dumbbells in front.

MIDDLE POSITION

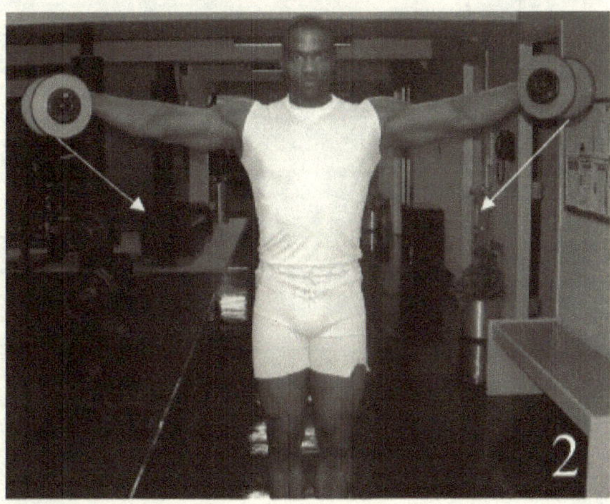

Raise the dumbbells evenly in a side lateral motion. Hold in that position for a second and contract your shoulders and trapezoid muscle at the middle point.

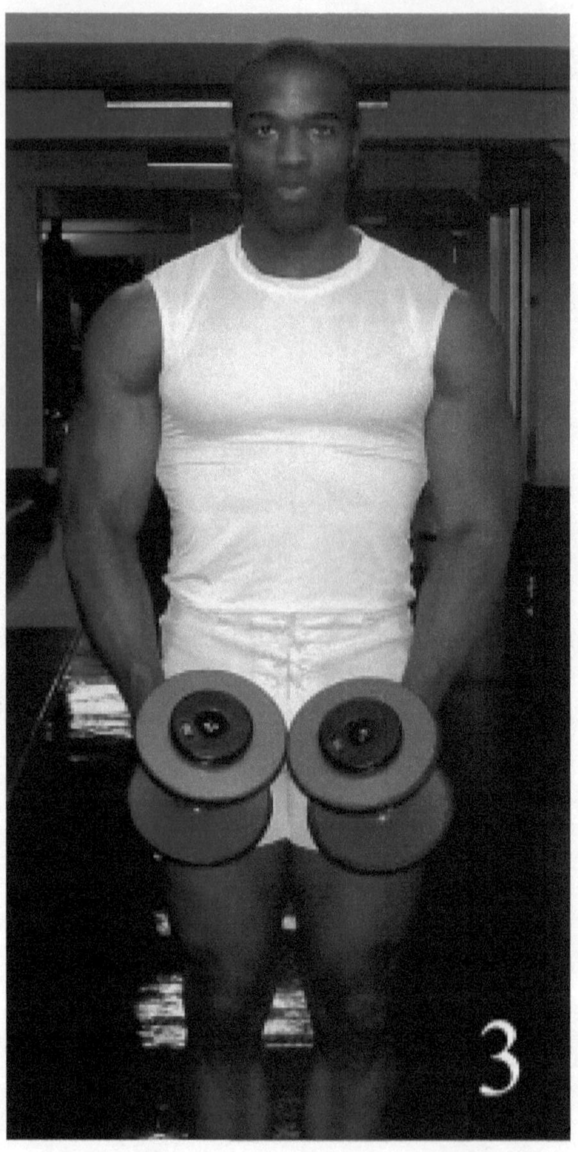

Lower the weight back to the starting position in a controlled manner and repeat this exercise for as many reps and sets desired.

Note: Keep your knees slightly bent and your back straight. As the weight is being raised upward, don't bend your back or lean backward, let your shoulders control the movement!

Shoulders (Barbell Upright Rows)

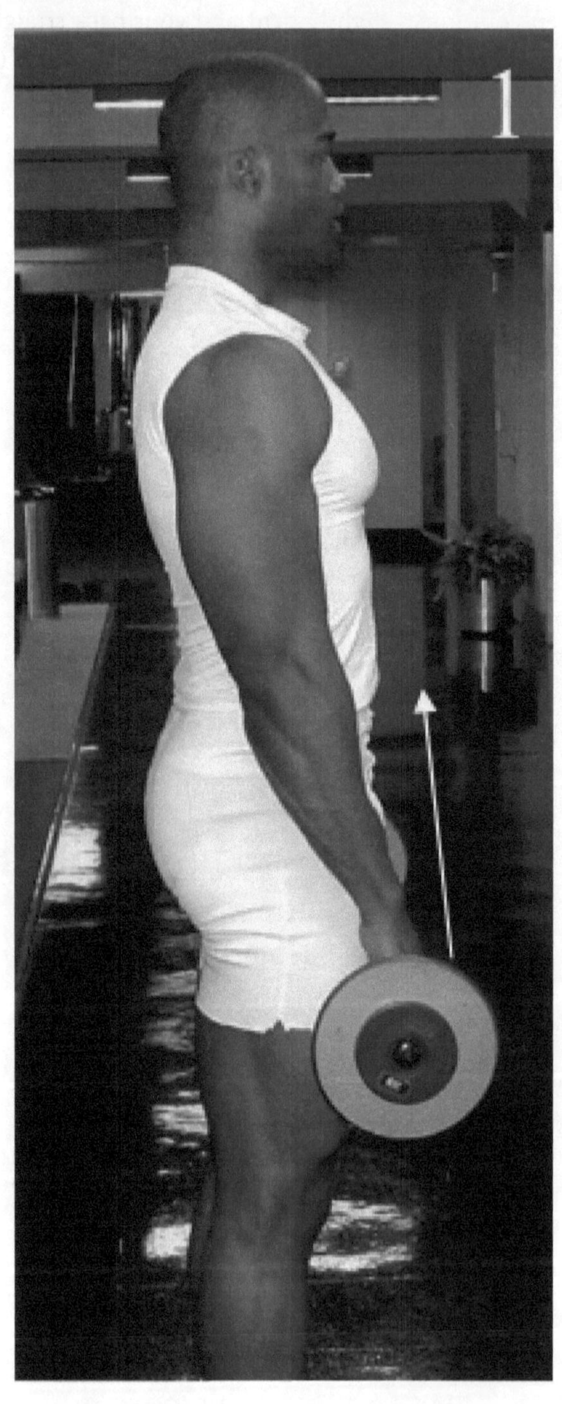
1

Measure your hands evenly on the barbell

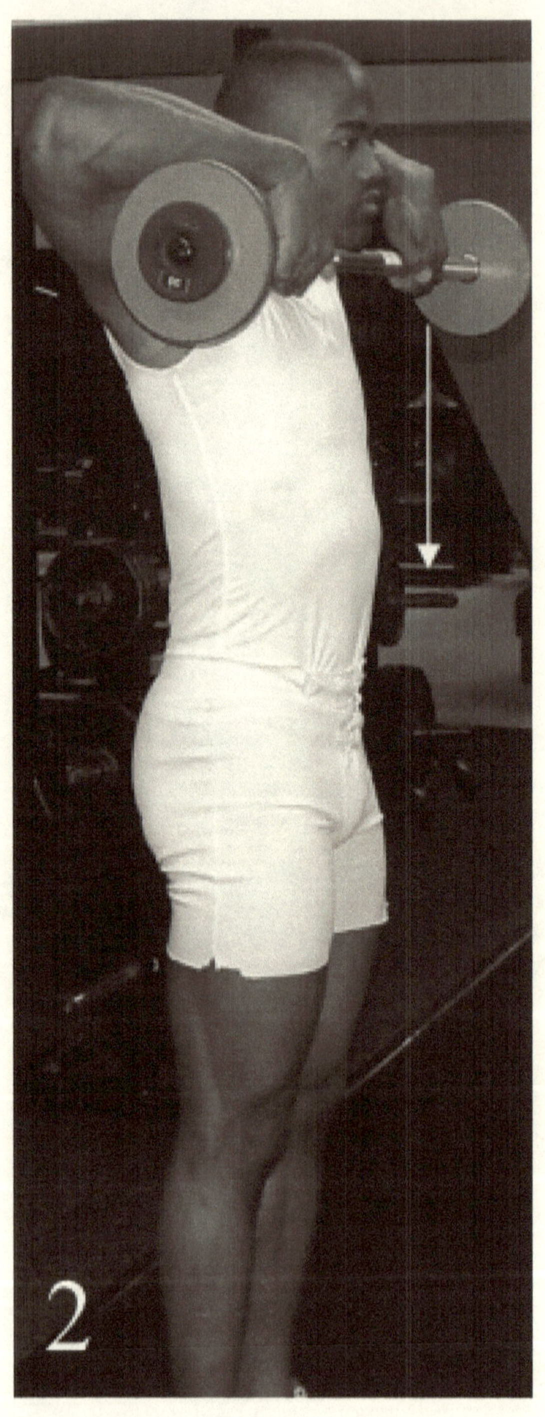
2

Raise the barbell upward towards your chin keeping your wrist relaxed so it can complete the motion. Inhale as you pull upward. Contract the Trapezoids muscles and hold this position for one second.

Note: My elbows must be higher than the shoulders, making sure they are even and on a straight line.

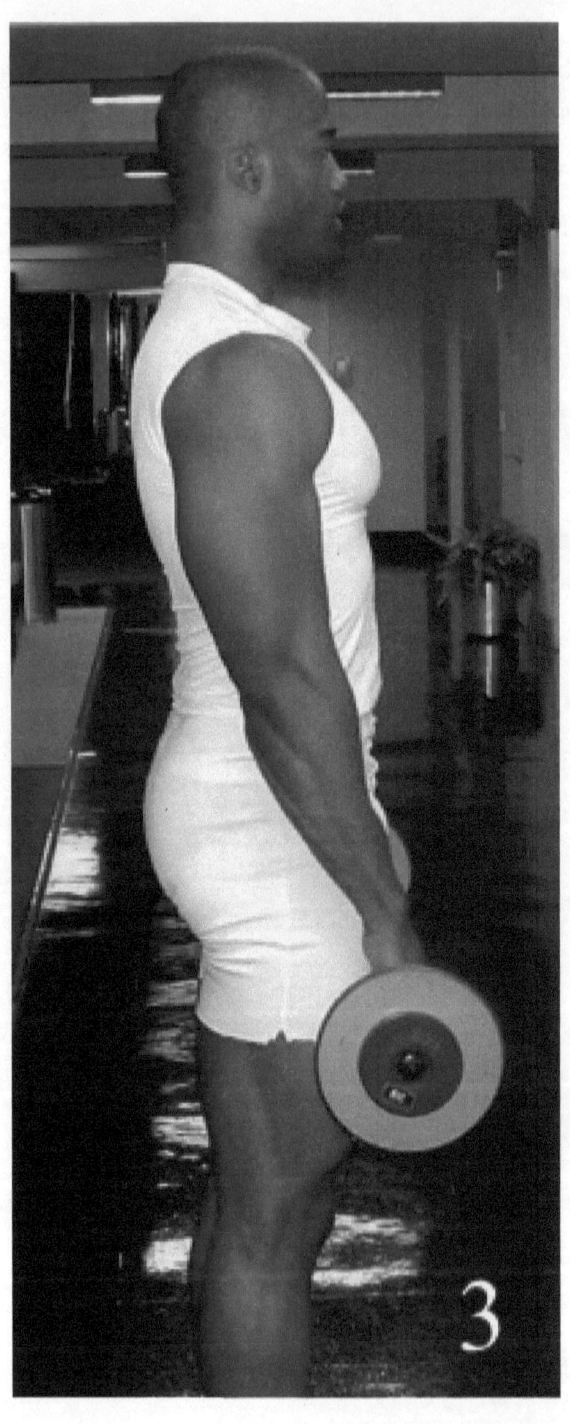
3

Exhale as the weight is lowered and repeat this motion for as many reps and sets as desired.

Note: Keep your knees slightly bent and your back straight. Don't lean backward, don't jerk or pull with your arms, use your shoulders, and raise your elbows head level as well. Let the motion remain smooth and fluid from start to finish.

Triceps (Cable push-downs)

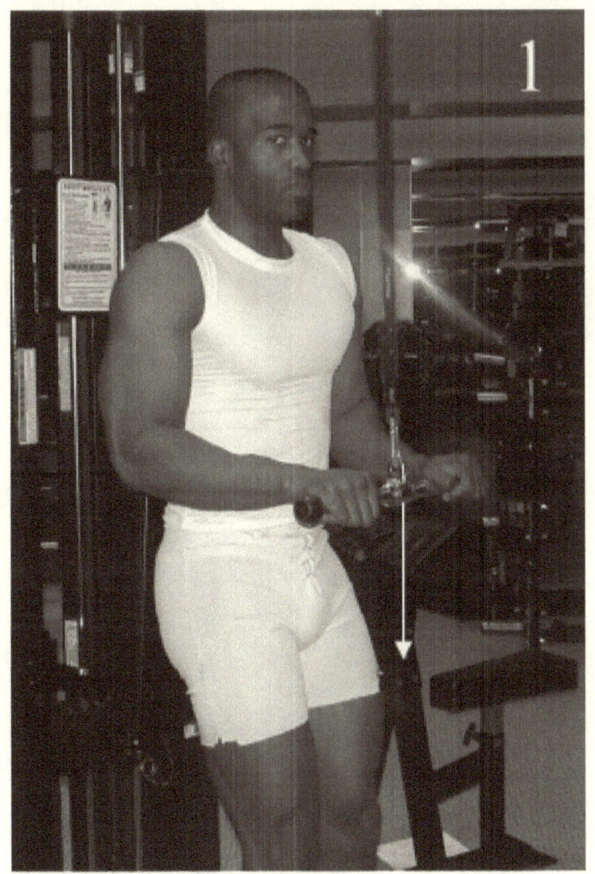

Make sure your hands are evenly placed on the bar. Start this exercise by getting your arms to a 90-degree position.

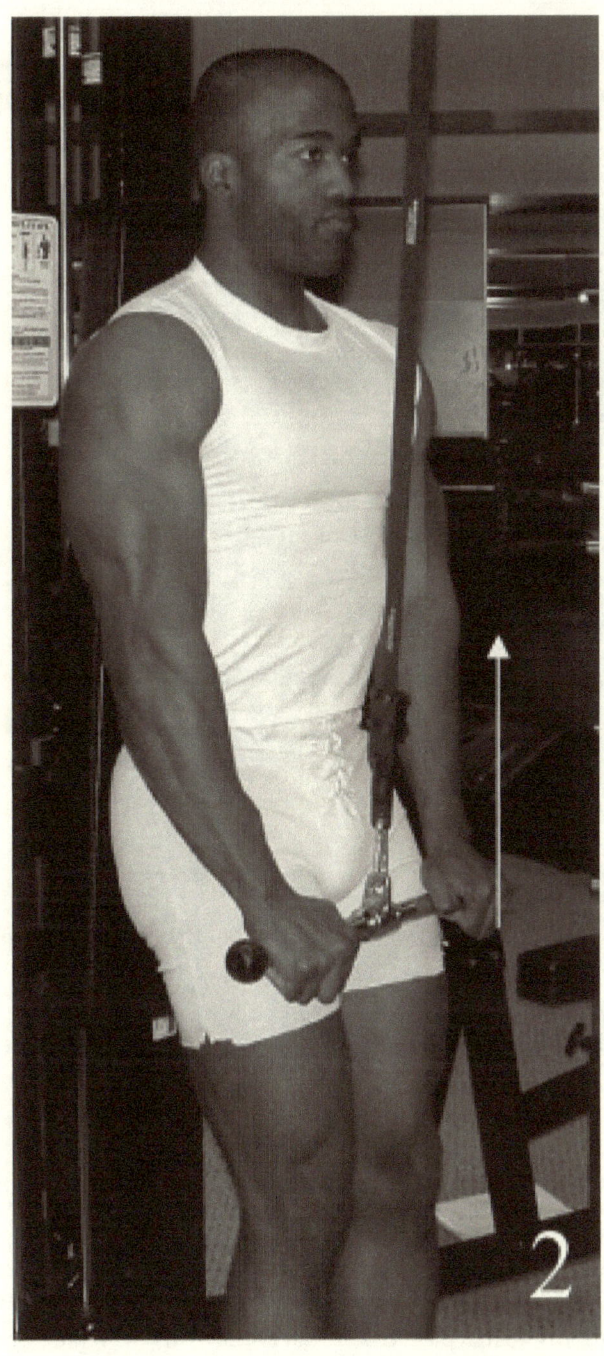

Push the weight towards your thighs contracting your triceps. Exhale as you push the weight and inhale as the weight is moving upward.

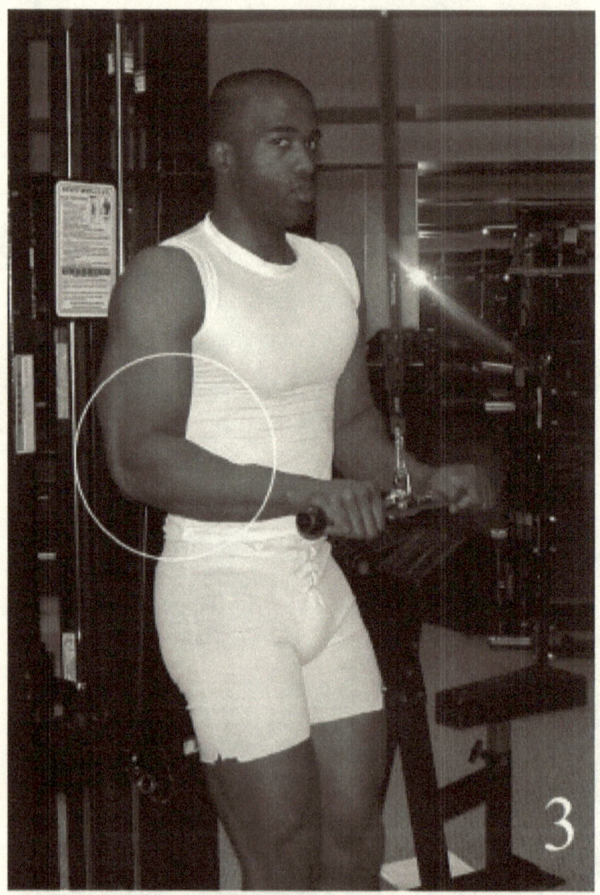

Return the weight back to the starting position (90 degrees) and repeat this exercise for as many reps and sets as desired.

Note: When my arm returns to the start position, the weight doesn't pull my arms past the 90 degrees. This will take the weight tension off the triceps and put the resistance on the shoulders. If you start to lean forward, lower the weight. ONLY YOUR TRICEPS should be trained in this motion. Make sure your back is straight and your knees remain slightly bent.

Triceps (Dumbbell kickbacks)

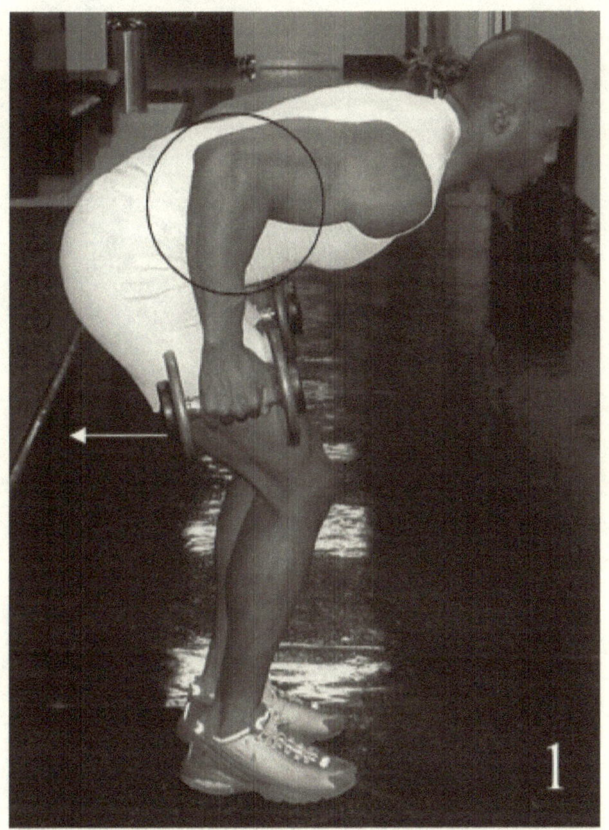

Bend your knees and make sure your back is straight bending your arm 90 degrees or horizontal to the floor.

MIDDLE POSITION

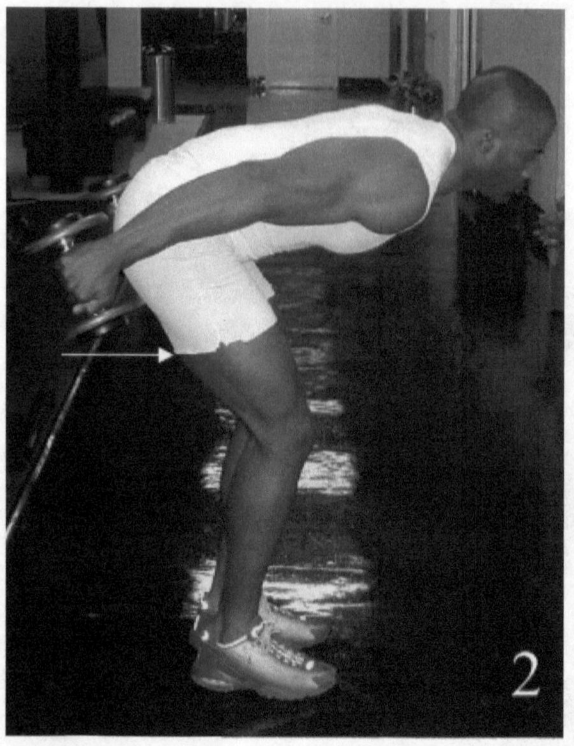

Push the weight in a backward motion holding the extension for one second.

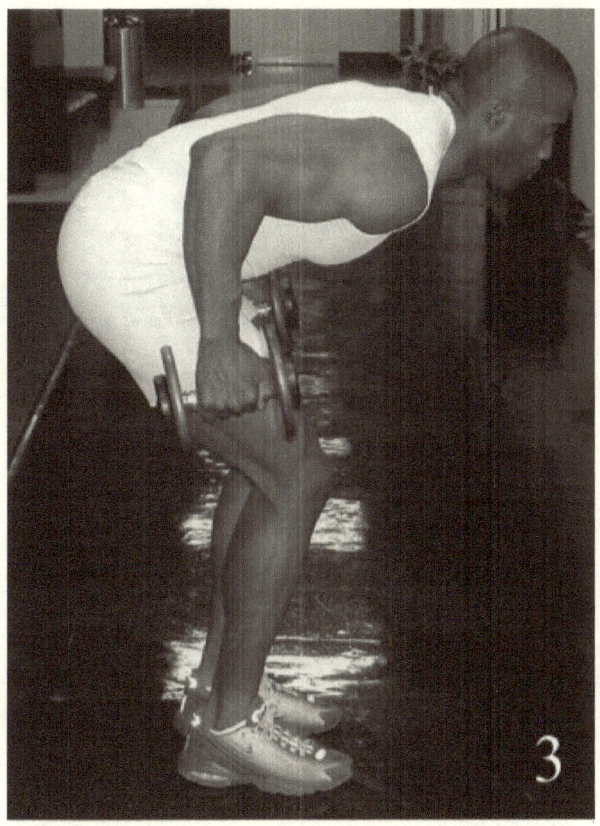

Lower the weight back to the start position, 90 degrees and repeat this exercise motion for as many reps and sets as desired.

Note: In the position of the body, there should be no swinging of the arms nor should there be any movement in the back to move the weight. Focus your efforts using your arms, mainly your triceps. Exhale on the pushing motion.

Back & Biceps (Lat Cable Pull Downs)

START POSITION

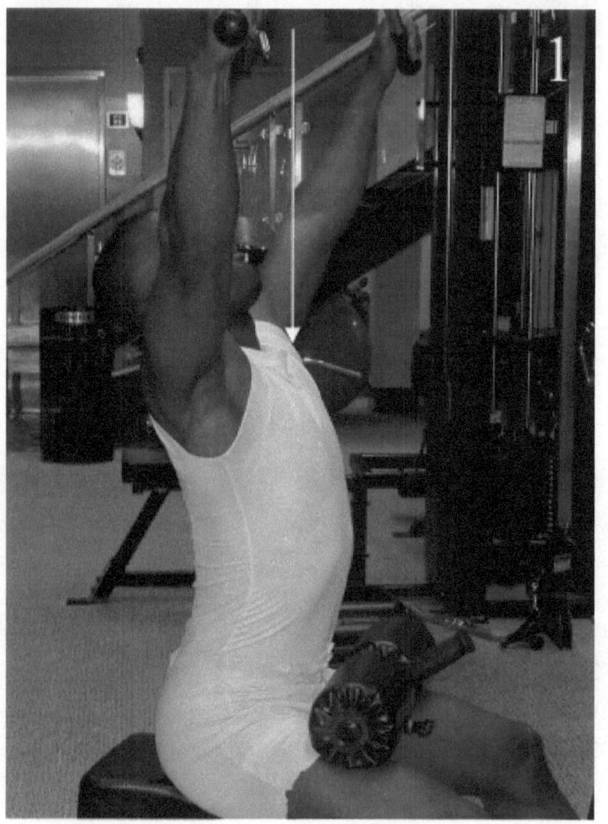

Secure your legs in the machine comfortably and make sure your
hands are measured even on the pull-down bar.

MIDDLE POSITION

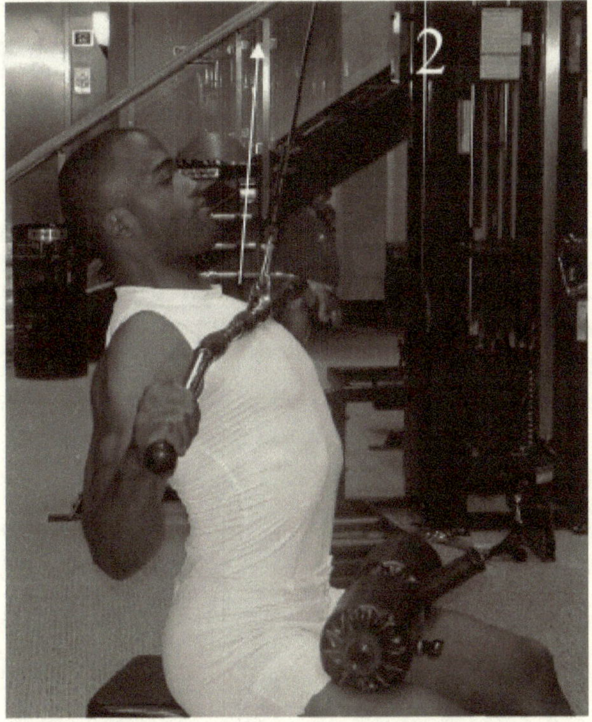

Inhale and make sure your back is straight and pull the load directly to the top of your chest. Contact your middle back in this motion for one second.

Note: The position of the arms in diagram 2. Also, there is no movement or leaning of the back in this exercise.

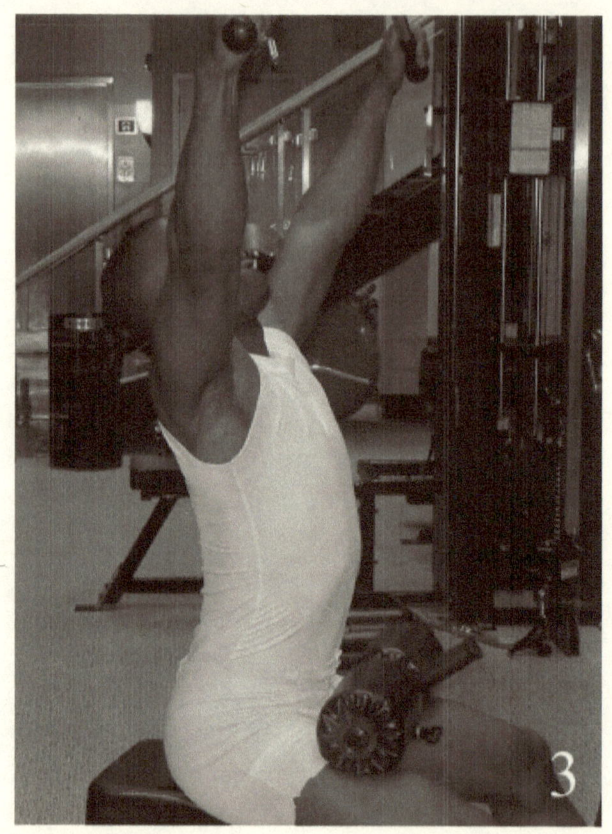

Raise the weight back to its start position and repeat this motion for as many reps and sets as desired.

Note: Exhale on the pulling motion. Make sure you don't jerk or bow your back on the downward motion. Focus on your upper and middle lats solely.

Back & Biceps (Seated Cable Rows)

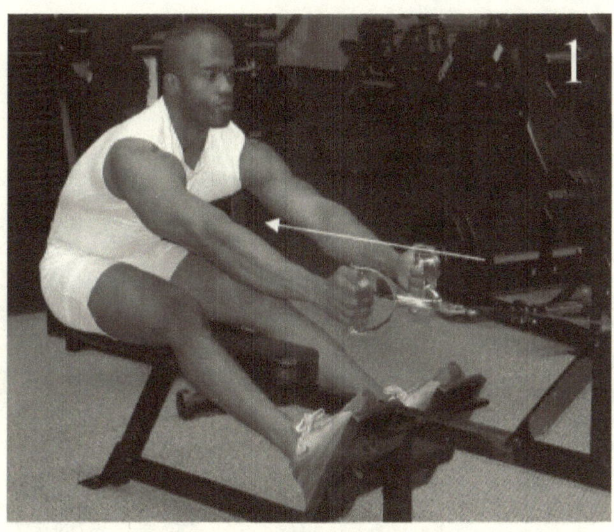

Make sure legs are bent slightly and your back is straight by poking your chest out and keeping your head up.

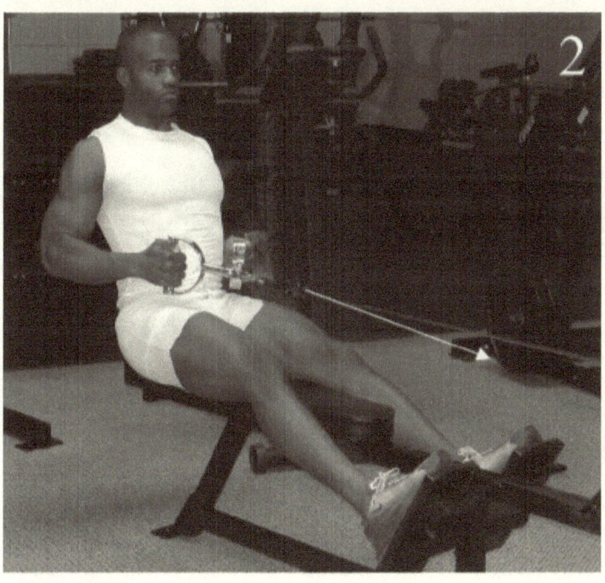

Pulling the weight towards your stomach keeping your elbows in a back position past your midsection. Exhale as you are pulling the weight. Hold the position for one second.

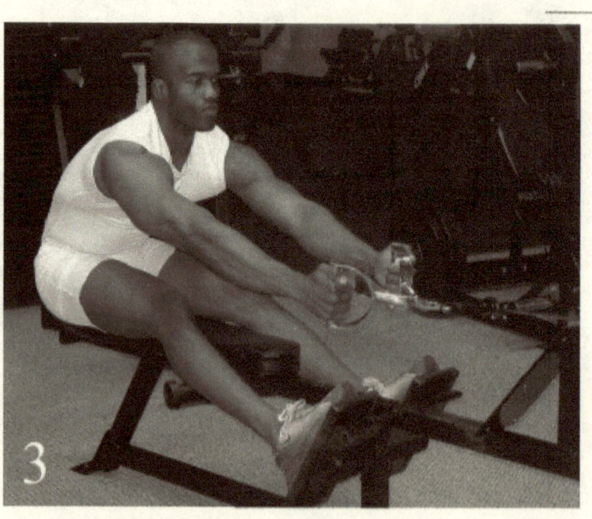

Return the weight back to the start position and repeat the motion for as many reps and sets as desired.

Note: There should be no jerking or snatching as the weight is being pulled to your stomach area. Make sure your back is straight throughout the entire movement. Don't let it curve or bow out at all!

Back & Biceps (Standing Barbell Curls)

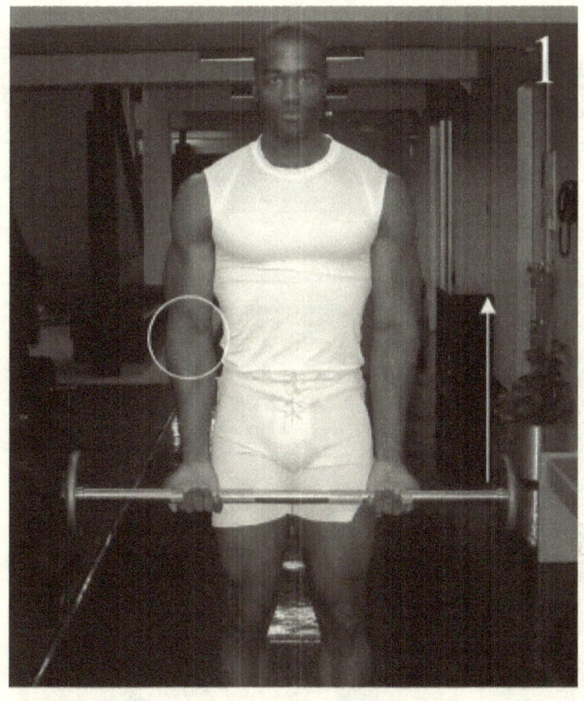

Keep your knees slightly bent and hands measured on the barbell.

MIDDLE POSITION

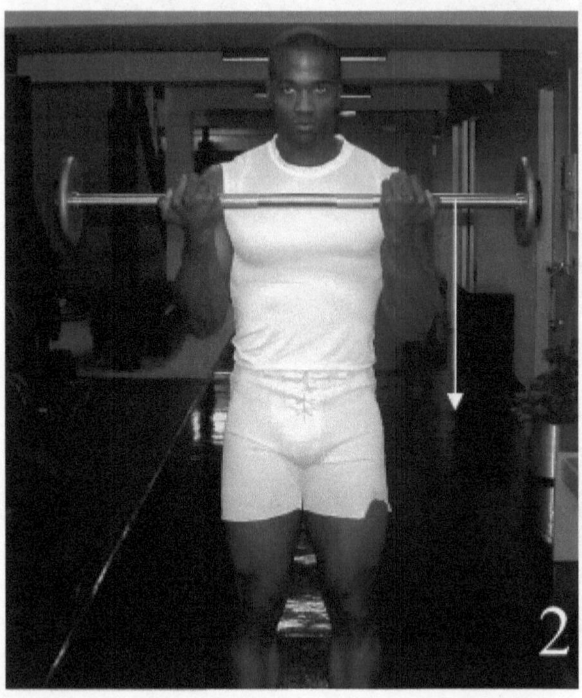

Exhale on the pulling motion upward and hold the position for one second.

Note: Let the elbows move in a natural motion, make believe you are squeezing someone's finger at the inner arm. See diagram 1 for a better biceps contraction.

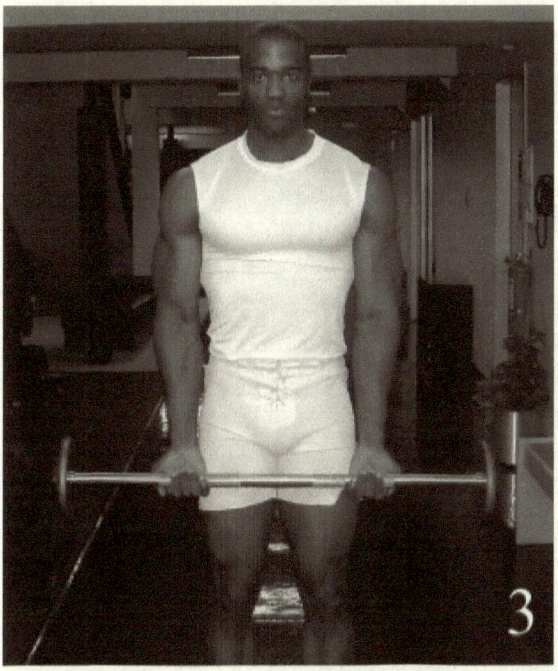

Lower the weight and repeat this motion for as many reps and sets as desired.

Note: Keep the motion focused on your biceps there should be no swinging of the weight or leaning backward of the back at all! This is dangerous and could cause lower back problems.

Legs (Barbell Squats)

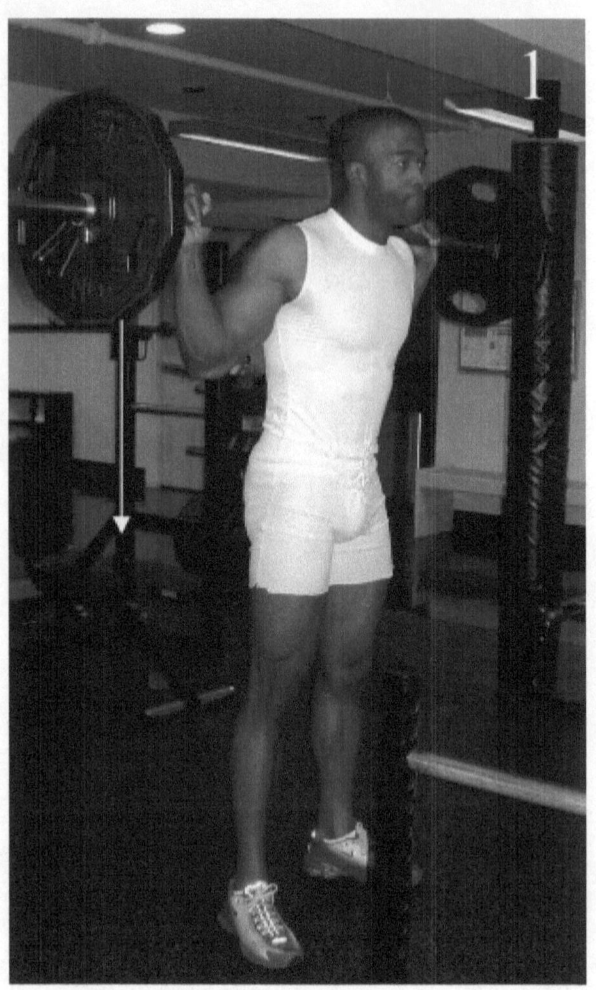

Start by placing your feet slightly past your shoulder line in a parallel
stance, your feet should be angled at 15 degrees.

MIDDLE POSITION

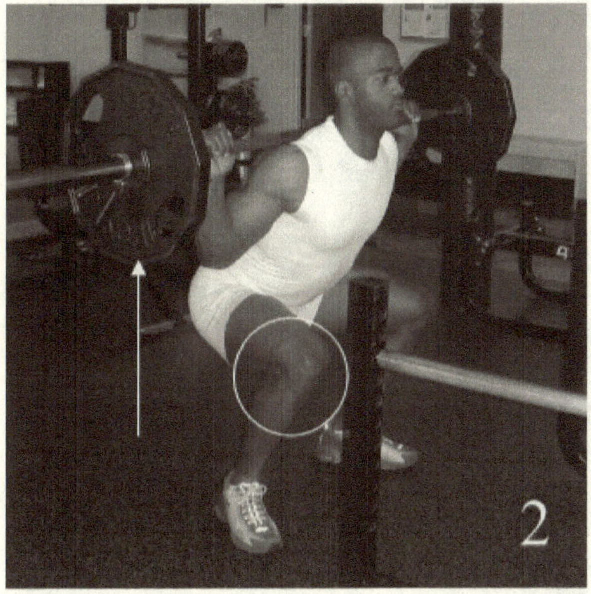

Start to release your waist first and then knees in a smooth squatting motion. See diagram 2.

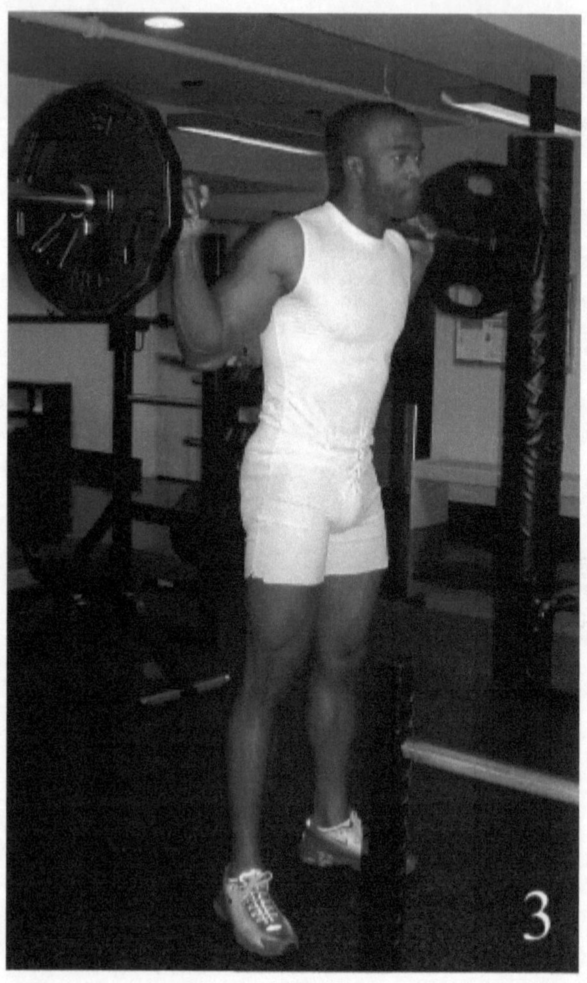

Exhale on the pushing motions. And repeat the motion for as many reps and sets as desired.

Note: Make sure the weight is balanced on your shoulders and keep your back straight by poking your chest out at all times. Keep the weight on your heels and push with both legs evenly. Never lock the knees at all as this will keep the resistance on the quads. Keep your head up at all times and don't hold your breath. Never go past 90 degrees in the squirting motion. See Diagram 2.

Legs (Seat Leg Press)

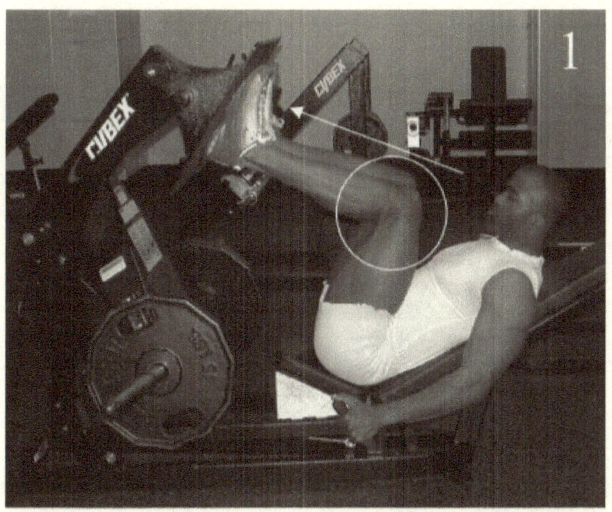

Measure your feet on the machine placing your feet slightly toward the top of the footplate.

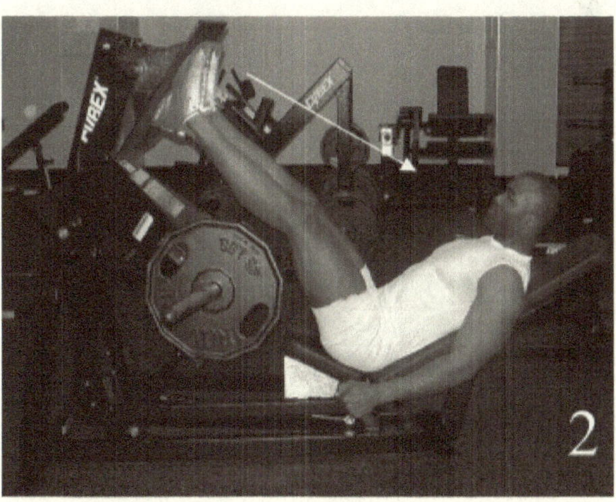

Release the weight and push the weight upward evenly with both legs.

NOTE: The knees should be at a 90 degrees position in the start and finish position. At the top of the movement contract the legs. DON'T LOCK THE KNEES IN THE RAISED POSITION. Keep your back on the pad at all times.

If your knees move past 90 degrees and your waist comes off the pad in the downward motion then you have gone too far in the motion. See Diagram 3.

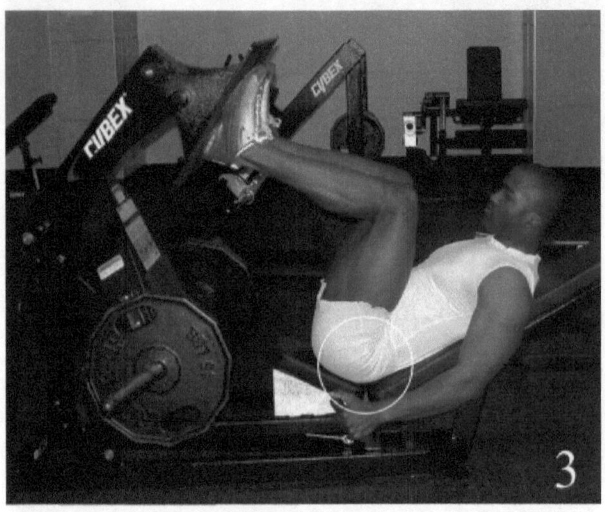

Return the weight back to the start position and repeat this motion for as many reps and sets as desired.

Legs (Leg Extensions)

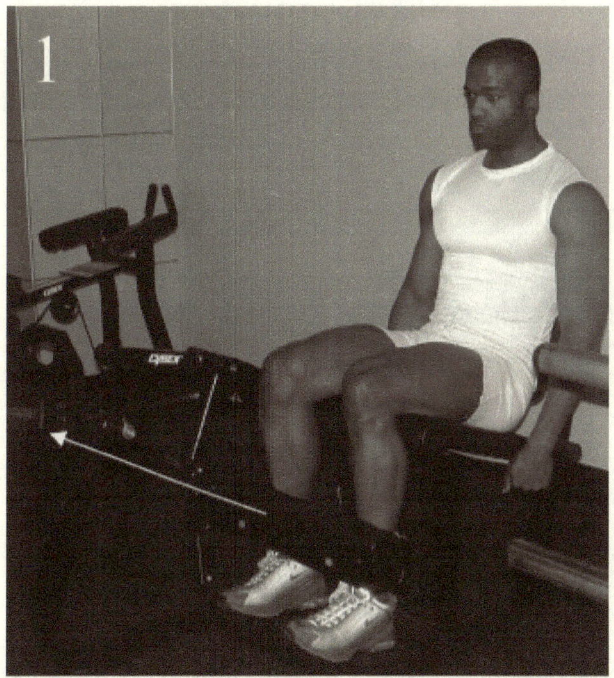

Sit in the machine and make sure the pad is placed comfortably at the top of your lower shins.

MIDDLE POSITION

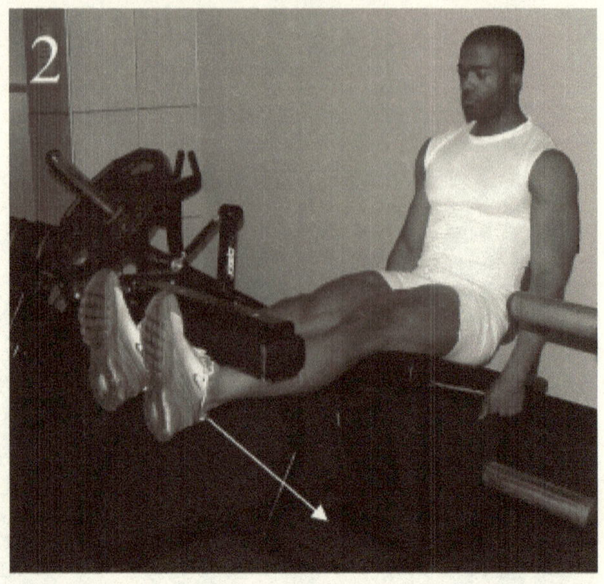

In a smooth motion, exhale and push the load upward. Contact the Quads and hold the position for one second.

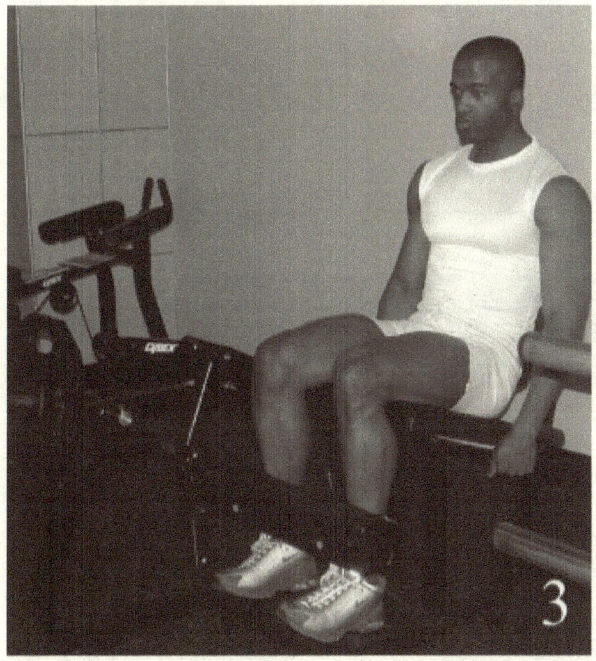

Lower the weight back to the start position and repeat the position for as many reps and sets as desired.

Note: Keep your butt on the pad at all times. Push the load in a smooth motion. There should be no jerking or rapid motion in the exercise.

Legs (Hamstring curls)

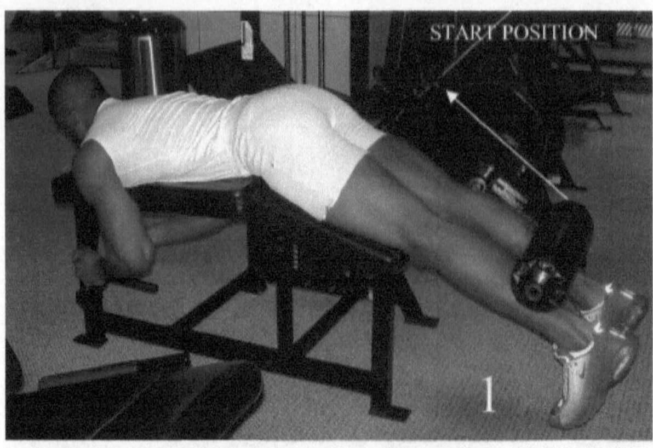

Make sure the pad is placed comfortably against your heels or lower calf.

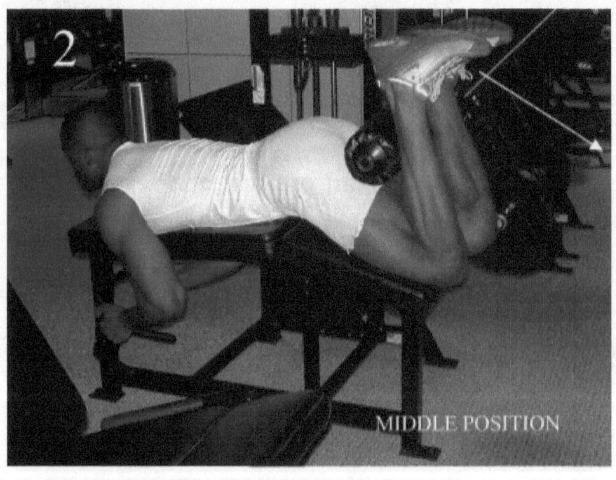

Use your hamstrings and pull the weight towards your butt holding this movement for a second.

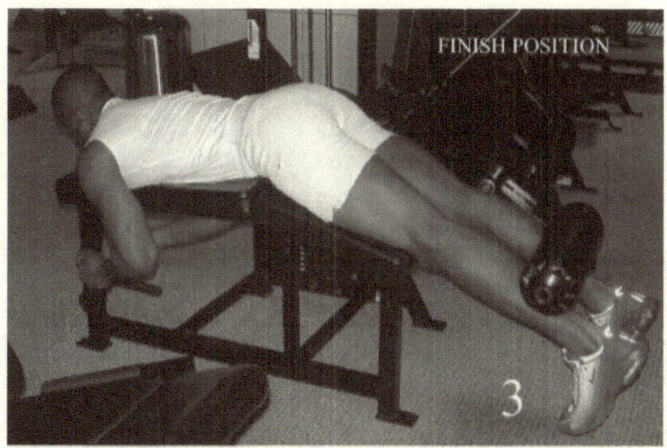

Lower the weight position and repeat his motion for as many reps and sets as desired

Note: Make sure you don't raise or lift your stomach off the pad. Breathe naturally and exhale on the pulling motions.

Legs (Stiff leg DeadLifts)

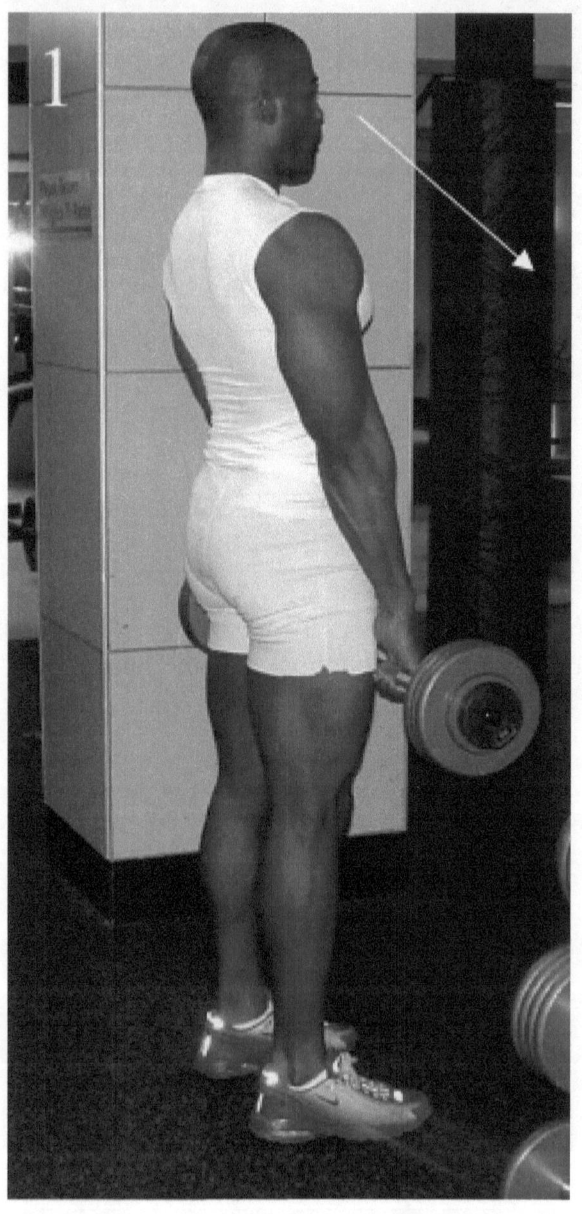

Make sure your hands are evenly measured on the barbell. Keep your

feet at shoulder width. Keep your back straight by poking out
your chest.

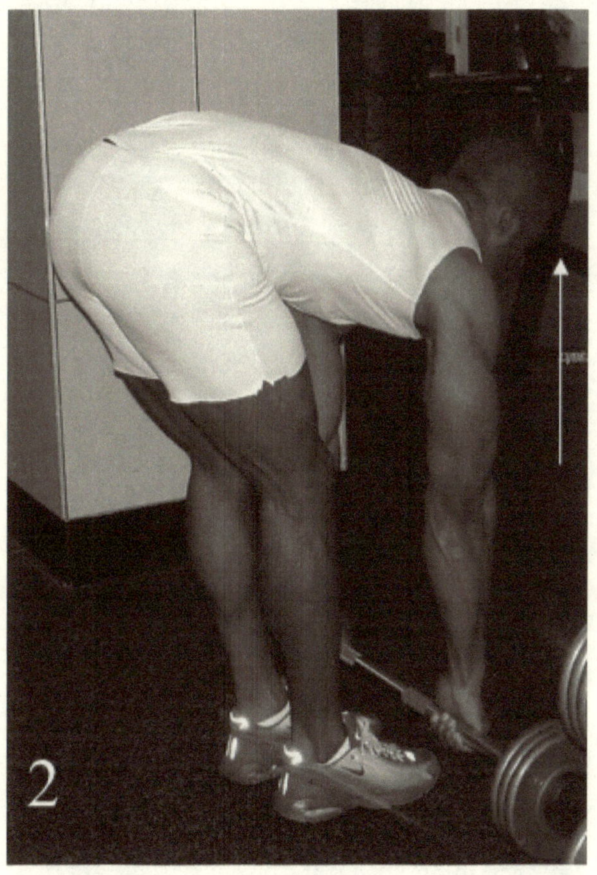

Release your waist and lower the weight towards your toes. Exhale on
the way down.

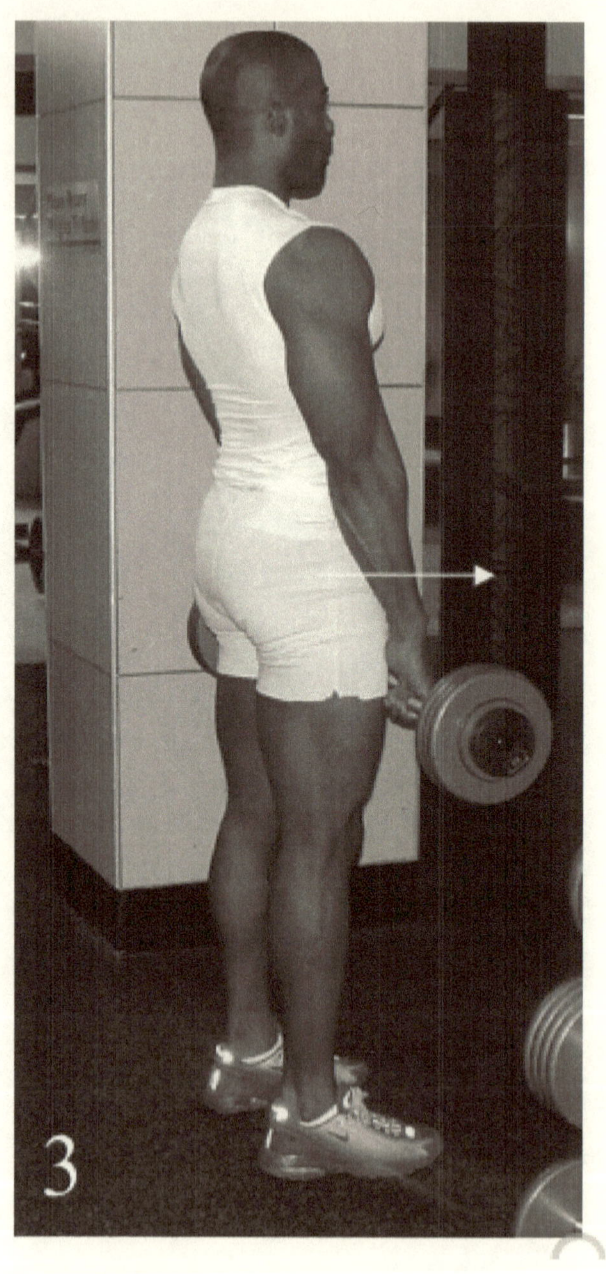

Keeping your back straight, use your hands to pull the weight upwards back to the start position. Push your waist in an upward movement.

Note: Keep your head up at all times while your knees stay slightly bent throughout this motion.

NATURAL BODYBUILDING DIET

Your nutrition is very important when building muscles. Exercises alone can't help build the desired muscles. Your diet during the exercise can either make or break your progress. Therefore, you should be careful about what you eat. To obtain the best muscle mass you need,

- Calorie: You must take more calories than the amount you burn in a day. You should take about 250 to 500 calories over your daily calorie requirement when doing the exercises. Taking more calories will result in excess fat gain.
- Lean Protein: You need sufficient proteins to provide you with the building blocks for the muscle tissue. You need to consume 0.8 to 1.2 grams/lb of proteins of your body weight in order to effectively build your muscles. After the workouts, you add an additional 0.2 to 0.25 grams/lb of proteins to help recover your muscles and gain more strength.
- Carbohydrates: You need sufficient carbohydrates to give your body the energy it needs in assembling the protein building blocks into muscle tissue. The amounts of carbs and fats you eat depend on personal preferences. Some people will feel better taking 100 grams of carbs daily while others may prefer higher than that.
- Dietary fats: The fats are essential for regulating hormones such as testosterone home that is required in building muscle mass. Most people take 0.35 grams/lb of fat per day or lower than that.
- Water: Water is very essential for your overall health. Taking a lot of water plays a bigger role in your growth.

Proper hydration of your body boosts your digestion, helps in protein synthesis, and removal of waste in your body.

Taking plenty of water ensures nutrients are properly absorbed in your bloodstream and muscles as well as moving byproducts out of your body.

Always maintain a clean eating habit. That is, eating more natural foods instead of processed foods. Always go for healthy foods for you to build lean muscles, stay energized, and healthy.

Natural supplements

You can add natural supplements to your diet to boost your energy. There are plenty of supplements in the market and if you're not careful, you can easily be misled.

If you're considering incorporating the supplements always do a thorough investigation on the supplement to ensure it doesn't have any of the banned substances.

Check whether there are any clinical studies conducted on the product you're interested in and the ingredients included. A good supplement should have research done on each of the ingredients in the product and the benefits of each of the products.

A good natural supplement shouldn't have any additives, artificial sweeteners, or any dyes.

NOTE: Natural bodyweight training doesn't require you to go to a gym, you can do the exercises at the comfort of your home. These forms of exercises can help you enhance your strength, speed, endurance and flexibility.

Anybody can do these simple steps from anywhere. Always follow the steps shown in this manual to ensure you're doing them correctly and targeting the right muscles! You can also incorporate weight lifting & resistance training to work on your muscles.

CHAPTER TEN: HOW TO ORGANIZE YOUR RESISTANCE TRAINING ROUTINE FOR BEGINNERS, INTERMEDIATE AND ADVANCE ATHLETES

Write down your plan and take it with you. A workout card or written plan of training will help you keep track of your workouts and allow you to see the progress you are making. This will also help with your compliance and keep you motivated. This sheet should include information regarding the order of the exercises you perform, the number of sets and repetitions, the date and difficulty of each exercise.

This information will keep your resistance training workouts organized. By recording the weights or machines you use for each workout, you will know how much weight to use for the next workout session. This will make your workouts more effective. Additionally, a workout card or plan helps to prevent injuries by allowing you to see how you should adjust the weight you are using each workout, by knowing how difficult the last workout was. This will help you avoid increasing your weights too quickly.

There are many different approaches to designing a resistance training workout. The type of exercise chosen and the order of the exercises are mostly a matter of personal preference. Keep in mind what we discussed earlier that you want to work larger muscles first. The guidelines I am suggesting are applicable to everyone and will give you a general outline that you can expand on your own or with the help of a certified strength and conditioning specialist or certified personal trainer. (Hint: Always train with some standard exercises like flat bench press or weighted free weights legs squats. Don't get too fancy, these standard exercises are called "standard" for a reason.)

There are 5 main components of a resistance training program that you need to consider. These are:

1. Choice of exercises
2. Order of exercises
3. The number of sets of each exercise
4. The amount of rest in between sets or exercises
5. The intensity of each set

These components can and should be manipulated to change your routine to avoid stagnation and boredom. First of all, always begin your workout with a short warm-up as outlined in Chapter 1: Getting Started and Chapter 2: Do I Really Need to Stretch?.

The exercises you choose to perform should work for the major muscle groups. These groups include chest, back (upper and lower), legs (front and back), stomach, and arms (front and back). For specific recommendations on exercises, consult each chapter on resistance training: Chapter Four: The Facts About Resistance Training for Women; Chapter Five: The Facts about Resistance Training for Men; and Chapter Six: The Facts About Resistance Training for Pre-Teen/Teen/Adults and see Sample Workouts at the end of this chapter. You will find exercises that not only cover each muscle group but that also come in different forms: body resistance, resistance bands, free weights, and weight machines.

You should perform 8 to 10 exercises that cover each of these muscle groups. (Meaning 3 sets of Quads, 3 sets of Hams, 3 calves and 1 set of Abs = a total of 10 max exercises.)

When you are choosing the order of your exercises, you want to perform the exercises that use multiple or large muscle groups first and then perform exercises that use single or small muscle groups next. Multiple or large muscle group exercises include the chest press, the bench press and the leg press. Single or small muscle group exercises include the biceps curl, the triceps pushdown, and the leg extension. This will allow you to maximally stimulate the larger muscle groups. (Note: Larger muscles normally push or press like legs or bench press, while smaller muscles pull Like Lat pulldowns and bicep curls).

When you are organizing your exercises, you may choose to alternate one body part with another of like working groups, meaning when you perform flat bench press for your chest, you are also using and warming up your shoulders and triceps which are the back of your arm. To add complete muscle overload, perform both a push and pull routine in one workout - like chest and back routines one after another with 'NO' rest. This order will allow you to rest one body part while you are exercising the other. Always perform the exercise throughout the full ROM (Range of Motion). This is important to help your muscles develop strength throughout their entire ROM and to keep them as flexible as possible. However, if you experience pain during some portion of the movement, you may need to use a pain-free or limited ROM. (Note: to perform a push-pull routine takes a lot of energy and you must work your way to that level, otherwise, you could injury yourself doing such movements due to rapid muscle fatigue. So don't expect to get to this point in your first few months of training. Be patient with yourself and make this your goal.)

The intensity of each workout is dependent on the number of sets you perform, the number of repetitions for each set, the weight you use, and the rest you take in between sets. Higher intensity workouts include doing more sets, decreasing the number of repetitions per set, increasing the weights used and decreasing the rest periods in between sets. However, if you do fewer repetitions with higher weights, you may need more rest to allow yourself to recover from the last set so you can be effective on the next set. The maximum rest should be 60 seconds or one minute. Lower intensity workouts include fewer repetitions, less weight, and possibly more rest in between sets. Although the rest can be shorter because you do not need as long to recover in between sets, since the intensity is lower.

To avoid boredom, you can change your exercises or the order of exercises whenever needed, or every 3 months. (Hint: Use light and heavy loads regularly within your training cycles to keep the muscle stimulated for maximum growth and strength gaining potential.) This will change the stimulus your body faces and make it constantly work to adapt to the new workout.

If you will be competing in Martial Arts, MMA, or other combat fighting, you will want to train like you're going to perform. That means that you need to have days of training as though you were in the ring fighting. Train intensely for 3 3-minute rounds working up to 5 5-minute rounds.

A good ending to a training session, before cool down, is to 'burn out'. Blast your cardio system, boost endurance to your muscles with intense low-weight vigorous work. This will completely fatigue the muscles. This encourages maximal glycogen depletion for muscle strength to increase. For example, hold a light dumbbell (1lbs) in each hand and jab, jab, jab, jab, jab as fast as you can until you can't hold your arms up anymore. Or for circuit work do it for 10 one minute sets. You should be bouncing lightly on your feet as you perform this thrust. Not every workout needs to end with a burnout. You can think of these 'burn out' sessions as a treat for your muscles.

You might try bicycles with ankle weights for a lower-body burnout. Lie on your back on a mat with hands clasped behind the head. Alternately bend each leg to the chest while twisting up at the waist to touch the elbow to the knee.

Here are several other ideas for an end of workout burnout.

Box Jumps

Start on a bench or other stable jump height platform. Jump down and the moment your feet touch the ground, launch back up to the starting place. Make sure you are fully balanced before repeating.

Try to reach 20 reps. If you fail, rest for five seconds and continue. Remember, this is a burnout. You are going to completely fatigue. Push yourself beyond what you think your limits are.

Cable Pushdown Tricep Finisher

With a fairly light weight, keeping the weights from ever clanging together (meaning the cables need to be under constant tension), press down *fast*. Hold for one second. Release up *fast*. Hold for one second. Repeat for 50 repetitions. If you fail before you reach 50, rest for 5 seconds. Then continue. This is a 'burn'. Keep at it. Push, push, push.

Rowing Machine Finisher

Use the actual rowing machine, not the cable rows on the weight machine. Do a 500-meter row as fast as you can. Rest for 3 minutes. Perform a 300-meter row followed by a rest of 2 minutes. Row all out for a 200-meter row. Then rest for 1 minute. Finally, power out your workout with a 100-meter row. You should be as limp as a wet noodle.

Drop Set Bicep Burnout

The dumbbell rack is already set up for you so let's use it like it is. The move is an Alternating Dumbbell Curl. Choose a weight at which you will fail at between 4 and 6 repetitions. For this example, let's say 40 lbs. In good form, with a dumbbell in each hand, stand straight and tall, feet shoulder-width apart and firm, core tight.

The curl is performed by swiveling the dumbbell parallel to the body with the palm of the hand facing away from you. Keeping the arm hanging parallel to the body with the action happening in the forearm through the contraction is in the bicep. Your elbow will move slightly forward to be just in front of your hips. Your body should remain firmly planted - it should not rock side to side as you perform this move. If it does, you are using momentum rather than muscle to move the weight.

Curl the right weight to the bicep with a firm exhale. Return to start. Repeat on the left. There will be no rest between these sets. Walk straight down the rack, dropping by 5 lbs. each time, regardless of where you start. Remember to start at a weight at which you fail at between 4 and 6 repetitions. The last drop in weight will be larger, dropping by 10 lbs. since you are clearly fatigued. But this is your last 'burn out' so you will do higher reps.

Let's begin:

- Do the curls with the first weight quickly (40 lbs. is our example) - 4 to 6 reps.
- Drop down the rack to the next weight - 35 lbs. for just 2 to 3 quick reps.
- Drop down to the next weight - 30 lbs. for our example. Perform another 2 to 3 quick reps.
- Drop down again - 25 lbs. Curl 2 to 3 times again.
- Drop down a larger weight this time - you're really feeling the burn. Let's go down 10 lbs., so we're at 15 lbs. for our example, and this time kill it with 4 to 6 reps. Wait. Got two more in you? Bang 'em out.

Plank Rows

Keep in mind you're performing a finisher. You're already fatigued. So the weight is low and the motion is quick.

You will do a plank over a set of dumbbells.

Keep your body straight and taut, core firm.

Draw one weight up towards the ribcage, bending your elbow. Lower back down.

Repeat on the other side.

Be sure to make repetitions quick. Shoot for 12. If you can pump out another few, do so. Your body will be shaking.

Kettlebell Swings

This begins in a deadlift position, only you're holding a kettlebell instead of a bar. Get a good grip on the kettlebell. Your next move is to swing the weight between your legs then explode it up to chest height where you are in a tightened core, upright plank position. Explode your breath in an exhale as you bring that bell to a stop at your chest. Arc it back down. You must maintain control of the kettlebell at all times. Bend your knees but do not squat. Shoot for 20.

Squat Sprawl

This is a hinge-like move. Stand with feet hip-width apart arms stretched overhead. Squat. Pivot hands to ground thrusting legs back into the plank position. Make sure your core is *tight*. Jump feet back to hands and push back up to the squat with arms swinging overhead. Hinge down to repeat. Aim for 10 but if you can kick out 2 more, more power to you. Seriously. You will be building more power in yourself.

Lunge Jumps

Starting in a lunge position, lower a knee to the ground. Jump up, switching arms and legs in mid-air (almost as though running in the air), then land softly, lowering to the opposite knee. That's one Lunge Jump. Shoot for 10, burning out a couple more if your mind doesn't stop you. You gonna let a little thing like a thought hold you back? Buck up buttercup!

Medicine Ball Slam Down

It's always great to vary the equipment you're using. While we're performing burnouts for our body, we don't want to burn out our gym routine and changing it up will keep us coming back for more. So let's add a medicine ball.

The medicine ball works for this exercise because its density keeps it from rolling away so we can easily recover it after slamming it to the ground.

Stand with feet - yep, you guessed it - hip-width apart, while holding a medicine ball. Lift the ball overhead as far as you can. Slam it to the ground. This is a hard, explosive, all-out move with as much power as you can. Land the ball in front of you so you can retrieve it, with a squat, in place. Repeat the movement. Perform fast and hard. Burn, baby, burn. Again, you're aiming for 10 reps but slam out a few more if you've got the least little bit of anything left in you.

Dumbbell Thrusters

For this one, you're going to use a heavier weight but remember you shouldn't be able to do too many reps.

In our standard stance of feet hip-width apart, place dumbbells (one in each hand) over your shoulders. Lower into a squat. As you raise, you will thrust the dumbbells into the air to full stretch. As you lower them back down to your shoulders, you will lower back down into a squat.

Burpee Squat Jumps

Start with feet shoulder-width apart. Drop to a burpee - hands to the ground, feet thrust back. Drop your chest to the ground. Touch your hands to the front of your head. Hands to the ground beside the chest. Pull your legs in while thrusting upwards. Jump into the air tucking your knees high, hands straight out in front. Repeat quickly as many times as you can. Can you hit 12?

REMEMBER, ALL OF THESE 'BURN OUT' exercises need to be done at maximum intensity with your full power behind them giving every effort you've got so that you 'burn out' the muscle to its final fatigue. These moves test your mental stamina as well as your physical prowess. You're already fatigued from your workout. Do you have the mental toughness to go the extra mile? To do the last bit of damage in the ring? To take down that opponent even though you feel like you can't lift your arms even one more time? That's what it takes to be a winner.

If you can push yourself through 'burn out' after your workouts, you'll be ready for that end-of-fight scenario. You'll have those reserves deep down inside of you and they will be ready for you to pull up in your time of need. But you've got to put them there first. The only way to do that is to train them into your body. Record them into your mind. Show yourself you've got the stamina, the inner strength to go that extra step, to blast out that last move, to pull up that one last ounce of reserve and crush it!

Now for some sample workouts. I've given you a couple of examples and started you on your way to a workout of your own. You now know that to avoid workout drop out, you need to keep things interesting. That means creating interesting workouts. These guidelines will help you get there. Remember to do these resistance training workouts with a rest day between. Those off days can be used to add even more interest to your workouts. Do something fun that you like to do - play soccer, horseback ride, ATV, run, mountain bike. You can think of lots of things. Or - here's a novel idea - rest.

Now let's get to the good stuff - the workouts!

SAMPLE WORK OUT #1:

Warm-Up

<u>Joint Rotations</u>

- Beginning at your fingers and working down to your toes (being sure to include the neck) or working from your toes upward, rotate each joint to stimulate the flow of synovial fluid (joint lubricant).
- Rotate joint clockwise and counterclockwise until movement is fluid and free
- Fingers
- Wrists
- Elbows
- Shoulders
- Neck
- Hips
- Knees
- Ankles
- Toes

<u>Aerobic warm-up</u> - choose one of the following: (Note: these are today's choice. There are lots and lots of other possible choices for tomorrow and all the days that follow. See how many days in a row you can change it up.)

- Jog in place, jog on a treadmill, jog moving forward.
- Dance the cha cha (this is actually an excellent groundwork move for protecting the groin in fighting). Interesting trivia tidbit: Bruce Lee was a champion Cha Cha dancer. He won the 1958 Hong Kong Cha Cha Championship. For added aerobic capacity, jab and weave. Hey, the cha cha and weaving are almost the same thing. Who knew?
- Stationary bike

Stretches

- Head rolls - half and full rotation
- Shoulder Rolls - forwards and backward
- Arm circles - small, medium, large. Forwards and then backward.
- Trunk rotations - both directions
- Standing Toe Touches Feet Together (we'll use a variation in the next workout)
- Standing Alternate Toe Touches Feet Apart
- Standing Hurdle Stretch
- Lunge Stretch
- Heel Drop Stretch

Work Out

Since this is our first workout, we're going to start with my go-to three (bench press, deadlift, squat) with emphasis on perfect form. You've already worked out your weight. Now let's work on form. Start with just a bar to make sure you've got the correct form for each lift movement before adding weight. Then you'll know you're performing it correctly. Have a trainer check out your moves to be certain you're doing it right. When you've got the form down, you're ready to add it to your work out.

Bench Press - 6 to 15 repetitions (your trainer has the final say)

- As you perform this move, you will engage your entire body. Your feet brace against the floor and every muscle tightens. You want to get every single little motor unit firing from your toes spread against the ground to your calves pressing down into it with your shins perpendicular to the ground directly below your knees. Your legs, buttocks, back, abs, everything, are all braced and tight, supporting those hardest working muscles in your chest and arms. Nothing is spared here.
- Squeeze your shoulder blades together and press your back into the bench to prepare for the lift as you're grabbing the bar with a straight wrist.
- Inhale. Exhale as you unrack the bar. Inhale.
- Slowly lower the bar on an exhale imagining you're bending the bar in an arc down towards your body. This allows your elbows to naturally flex in to protect your shoulders by engaging your lats.
- Touch your chest and mentally prepare for the explosion of the push by pulling all the power of the room into your body and bracing.
- Press against the floor with your legs, your back arches slightly, as you burst up through your chest wall with an exhale to push the weight back up.
- Repeat for the appropriate number of reps.
- Rest for 3 minutes.
- Perform the next set. We'll be working towards a goal of 3 sets.

Deadlift

- You need a good strong stance for this. Layne Norton, PhD (IFPA & NGA Natural Pro Bodybuilder; Physique, figure, and bodybuilding coach; professional powerlifter) recommends a stance "where you would be able to jump the highest in a standing leap."
- Hinge at your hips to grasp the bar just to the outside of

your shins. Any further apart and you run the risk of injury.

- Remember, once again, that you are dealing with an entire body move. Fortify yourself for the move by inhaling and bracing your abdominals. This protects your spine for the lift, enabling you to generate maximum force.
- Engage your lats first - the large muscles of your back. This also helps prevent injury.
- The Pull: You are going to push your legs into the ground as you pull the bar as though bending it (as in the bench press) in a U towards yourself. Squeeze your glutes (your butt) and thrust your hips forward straightening your spine and firming up your entire body, especially your back. Think of the move as a pull to erection and a push through the floor rather than a lift.
- To lower, release your glutes and let your hips drive back creating a controlled fall of the bar to the floor. If you try to lower the bar too slowly, you risk torquing your back and causing injury.
- Repeat 6 to15 times with your trainer having the final say.
- Rest for 3 minutes.
- Next set. Again, we will be working towards a goal of 3 sets.

Squats

- Stand as though at attention; spine in alignment, head, and shoulders back, head raised, slight curve to the back. Your back will remain straight as the movement is in the hips. Also, your head will remain in alignment with your spine. No looking up. So far so good?
- Step up to the bar and get a comfortable grip. The bar should rest just above or below the sharp ridge of your scapula (shoulder blade). Your feet should be comfortable shoulder-width apart.
- Turn your toes out - about 45 degrees.

- Keeping your knees in line with your feet, and your abs contracted, engage your whole body as you 'sit' back as though going for a chair behind you.
- Lower to parallel to ground. An advanced trainee may continue to a full squat all the way to the ground. Be sure you have thoroughly stretched your ankle tendons so as not to tear them.
- Reverse immediately by driving back upwards. The ascent should be squeezing your glutes together, pulling your hips in as hard as possible, as though a giant were pulling you from the front of your hips and the back of your neck to try to straighten you out.
- Breathe. Repeat.
- Your goal is 6 to15 repetitions.
- Rest for 3 minutes.
- Repeat the set. Try to reach 3 sets.

Burn Out

<u>Squat Sprawls</u>

Squat sprawl 'til you can't move. If you can do 10, you're amazing. Pump out more for superhero form.

Post Workout Stretch

<u>Lunging Hip Flexor</u>

- On the ground, have one knee bent with the foot flat on the ground. Kneel on the other leg.
- Lean forward to stretch the front thigh and hip of the kneeling leg.
- Hold the stretch for 30 seconds.
- Switch legs.

<u>Piriformis Stretch</u> - this is the muscle that runs from your spine to your hip.

- Sitting on the mat or ground, stretch both legs before you.
- Bring one leg in across your lap, placing your ankle above your knee.
- Lean slightly over your leg until a stretch is felt in the buttocks.
- Hold for 30 seconds.
- Switch legs.

<u>Abs Stretch</u>

- Rollover to your stomach. Stretch out.
- Place your hands on either side of your chest.
- Push slowly upwards-arching up and stretching out your abdominal muscles.
- Hold for 30 seconds.

<u>Chest Stretch</u>

- Sitting or standing, grasp your arms behind your back with fingers interlocked.
- Gently press arms back and away from the body contracting shoulders together to open up the chest.
- Hold for 30 seconds.

SAMPLE WORK OUT #2:

You've rested a day since your last work out, let your muscles recuperate. You've participated in your other sports but you haven't done any more resistance training. Today, we're back at it. Ready to pump it up.

Warm-Up

<u>Joint Rotations</u>

- Beginning at your fingers and working down to your toes (being sure to include the neck) or working from your toes upward, rotate each joint to stimulate the flow of synovial fluid (joint lubricant).
- Rotate joint clockwise and counterclockwise until movement is fluid and free
- Fingers
- Wrists
- Elbows
- Shoulders
- Neck
- Hips
- Knees
- Ankles
- Toes

Aerobic warm-up - choose one of the following: (Note: these are today's choice. There are lots and lots of other possible choices for tomorrow and all the days that follow. See how many days in a row you can change it up.)

- Jab and weave or shadow box
- Jump Rope
- Jumping Jacks

Stretches

- Head rolls - half and full rotation
- Shoulder Rolls - forwards and backward
- Arm circles - small, medium, large. Forwards and then backward.
- Trunk rotations - both directions)
- Lying Toe Touches Feet Together
- Lying Alternate Toe Touches Feet Apart
- Sitting Hurdle Stretch
- Deep Knee Bends

- Seated Calf Stretch with a resistance band

Work Out

Today we're going to use bodyweight resistance.

- Push-ups - or any variation to challenge you. See Chapter Five: The Facts About Resistance Training for Men for lots of interesting variations you can try. 6 to15 Repetitions. Rest for 1 minute.

You now have a choice of continuing through the rest of the work out then coming back to repeat each move for a second set, proceeding through all moves, then coming through for a third set. Or: do a second set of push-ups. Rest. Do a third set of push-ups. Then move on to Mountain Climbers. The choice is yours.

- While we're in this basic position, Mountain Climbers. Do 6 to15 Repetitions.
- Burpees. Perform 6 to 15 Repetitions
- Leg Raises. Repeat for 6 to 15
- Donkey Kick Back. Do 6 to15 Repetitions.
- Medicine Ball Sit-Up Throw
- Lay flat on your back with knees bent, medicine ball in your hands stretched out past your head.
- Explode your arms upward as you sit up and throw the ball forward.
- This is best done with a partner who can return the ball to you.
- Perform 6 to 15 Repetitions

Burn Out

As long as you've got the medicine ball out, do the medicine ball slam down.

- Medicine Ball Slam Down - Stand with feet - yep, you guessed it - hip-width apart while holding a medicine ball. Lift the ball overhead as far as you can. Slam it to the ground. This is a hard, explosive, all-out move with as much power as you can. Land the ball in front of you so you can retrieve it with a squat in place. Repeat the movement. Perform fast and hard. Burn, baby, burn. Again, you're aiming for 10 reps but slam out a few more if you've got the least little bit of anything left.

Post Workout Stretch

<u>Shoulder Joint Stretch</u> - After all those Slam Downs, you really need to loosen up your shoulders with this one.

- Hold a towel or resistance band between your hands with your arms stretched out in front of you
- Raise your arms up and up over your head until they are as far back as they can go.
- Resist arching your back.
- Hold for 30 seconds before returning to start.
- Repeat several times.

<u>Groin Stretch</u> - Also called 'Butterfly'

- Sit with your feet together, heels close to your groin.
- Press down gently on knees with your elbows to stretch.
- Hold for about 30 seconds.
- This stretch will be felt in the groin, glutes, hamstrings, and even the lower back.

<u>Forward Bend</u>

- This is like a standing toe touch only seated.
- On a mat or the ground, bend over your legs and reach for your toes.

- Touching your toes is not important.
- Simply stretch towards them feeling a gentle stretch all along the back as well as the back of the thighs and calves, even the arms.
- Inhale.
- As you exhale, relax your muscles into the stretch.
- Hold for at least 30 seconds.

DESIGN YOUR OWN WORK OUT:

You're going to follow the same pattern we've already set.

Warm-Up

Joint Rotations - These never change. All your joints need to be warmed up, every time.

- Beginning at your fingers and working down to your toes (being sure to include the neck) or working from your toes upward, rotate each joint to stimulate the flow of synovial fluid (joint lubricant).
- Rotate joint clockwise and counterclockwise until movement is fluid and free
- Fingers
- Wrists
- Elbows
- Shoulders
- Neck
- Hips
- Knees
- Ankles
- Toes

Aerobic warm-up - You'll determine this. Pick something you like. It needs to get your blood moving and bring your body temperature up a couple of degrees to prepare your body for stretching. This will take 3 to 5 minutes.

Write your choice down here:

Stretches - Start with these and then proceed down your body with stretches you choose. Write them in as you go. I've left the room.

- Head rolls - half and full rotation
- Shoulder Rolls - forwards and backward
- Arm circles - small, medium, large. Forwards and then backward.
- Trunk rotations - both directions)
- Your stretches:

Workout - Your biggest decision. In Sample Workout 1, we did the big three (Bench Press, Deadlift, Squats) using free weights. In Sample Workout 2, we did a body resistance workout. You could choose to do one of the workouts we haven't done yet - resistance bands or weight machines. Or choose to repeat one of the earlier types of workouts using exactly the same routines or entirely new resistance moves. Or, you could choose to do a combination of any of these. The field is wide open. Just keep in mind that today is resistance training. Work your larger muscles first. And follow a push exercise with a pull exercise.

Write your plan down here including the weight you plan to lift (even if it's body resistance) and how many reps and sets of each you intend to do:

Burn Out - Now finish off your work out with a good burn out. Remember, not every work out has to finish with a burnout. But if you can, go that extra mile. Do it now. Push it, push it, push it. Eat or be eaten.

What's your killer choice today? Write it down here:

Post Workout Stretch

Cover the areas of the body that you worked the hardest and then gently stretch your other muscles. Write them down here before you start your work out so you know what you will need to do. I've left you space:

You've just finished a killer workout you designed yourself. Congratulations! The only bad workout is the one you *didn't* do.

NOTES: Whether you're a beginner or advanced athlete, you have to organize your exercises based on what part of the body to work on. You should always consider the choice of exercises, the order to do them, how many sets or reps to do in each exercise, and the rest time between each set of the exercise.

You can switch the exercises to avoid being bored by having the same routine of workouts every day!

CONCLUSION

Martial Arts Notes

Resistance Training & Martial Arts

The American College of Sports Medicine has published guidelines for healthy individuals for the quantity and quality of exercise. Their recommendations are designed to develop and maintain cardiorespiratory and muscular fitness, as well as flexibility.

Their recommendations include:

1. Frequency of exercise: 3 to 5 days per week.
2. The intensity of exercise: Their recommendations are based on your "all-out effort" physical potential and are quite technical. For those familiar with the terms maximal heart rate, VO2 max, and HR reserve, the numbers are 55 to 90% of maximal heart rate and 40 to 85% of VO2 max or HR. The lower levels are intended for those who are "out of shape." As you continue to train, your maximal effort will obtain better and better results and your body will

become more and more conditioned and efficient. This means that with less energy, you will be able to do more.

3. Recommended duration: 20 to 60 minutes of continuous or intermittent bouts of aerobic activity accumulated during the day. Your total amount of aerobic exercise is what is important, not that it is done all in one session. However, 10 minutes minimum time per session is needed to achieve benefit.

4. Mode of activity: any activity qualifies that uses large muscle groups that can be maintained for a prolonged period, and is rhythmic and aerobic (using oxygen and elevating your heartbeat) in nature.

5. Rate of progression: In most cases, the conditioning effect (a lower heart rate and perception of effort) allows people to increase the amount of work they do per exercise session.

This is not competition level training. This is merely what's recommended to stay physically fit. You are going to want to train specifically for your sport, including the exercises and recommendations in this book, to progress in your fitness level, strength, and endurance in order to build up to competition level fitness.

FINAL WORDS

I've thought long and hard about how I want to conclude this book. What is it I want you to walk away with? Resistance training is an important part of any fitness program because it provides strength not just to your muscles but also to your bones. Just the fact that it contributes to the prevention of osteoporosis should be a motivating factor for anyone to make it a part of their regular health regimen. As young people, you're not thinking about that. But you should be. Fitness needs to be a daily part of your life from your earliest days. For all the many benefits it provides to you.

Gym dropouts are as high as 50%. Obesity is at 42.2%. That's up 3% from 2018 and 6% from 2016. We're in a crisis. Get up off that couch and save yourself from an epidemic.

There are so many ways that resistance training benefits your life. It not only helps you perform better at your chosen sport. It improves your everyday quality of life because it improves your strength and coordination. It makes everything you do easier, from flying kites to walking the dog. From fierce soccer kicks to enduring mountain climbs. White water rafting to something as simple as a leisurely walk through the forest. Shoot, even sitting around for an afternoon of video games is made easier when your body is fit from regular resistance training because the superior posture it provides keeps you from fatiguing as quickly as your less-fit counterparts.

You picked up this book. And hopefully, you've read it. So you're on the right track. Now implement it. Read the motivating affirmations. Study the workouts. Then get out there and put these methods into action. Your body deserves every bit of effort you put into it. You are the effort you put into you. Be stronger than your excuses. Start today. Right now. Put this book down. Put on your gym shoes and start lifting. Start with your own body weight. Right now. Drop to the floor and do your first plank. You've got this!

If you have enjoyed my book and the content was helpful please support this book by providing a review.

ABOUT THE AUTHOR

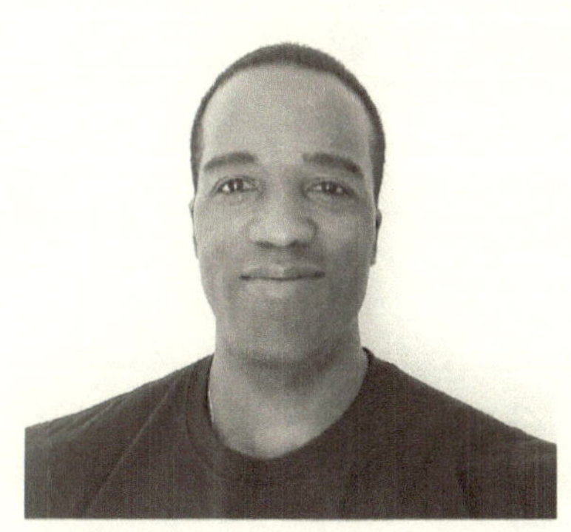

G.E.S. Boley Jr. – He is a devoted full-time father, husband, and Family Man who places Jesus above all else. George is a Martial Artist, Martial Arts Instructor with Multiple Black Belts in Taekwon-Do and Hapkido. George was a TaeKwon-Do National Sparring Champion and a Member of the 2007 USA Team. He is a Defensive Tactical Training Instructor, with training in hand to hand combat, stick and knife fighting and Freestyle Grappling. He is a health and fitness instructor and trainer, certified sports nutritionist, business entrepreneur, real estate investor, property manager, business consultant, and coach.

Along with training certifications, George has a Bachelor's Degree in Marketing and an MBA in Business. George has many life experiences and is passionate about learning and helping people in need.

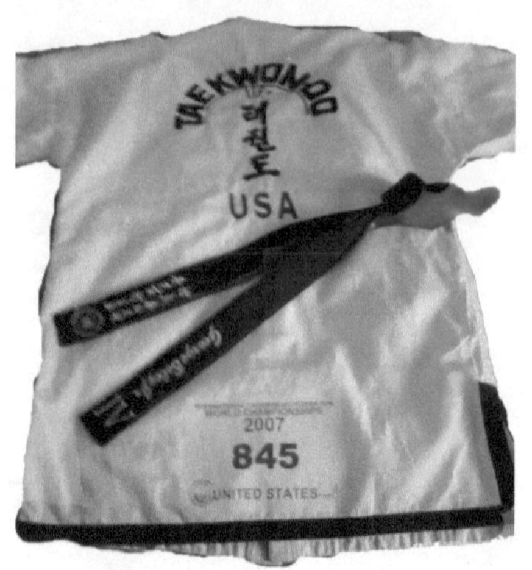

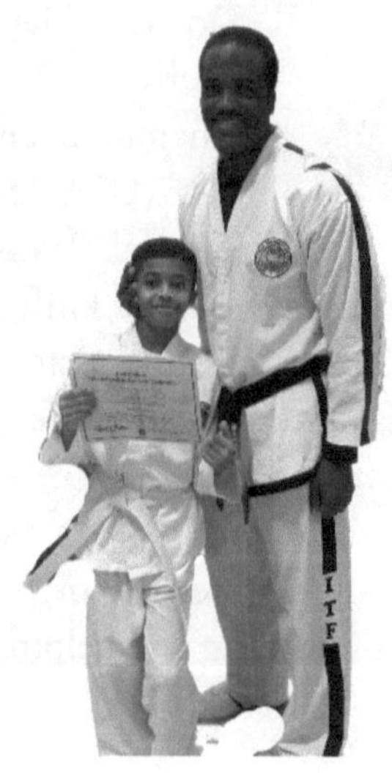

Yes, 100% FREE!

If you want insider access plus this Fitness Test Guide, all you have to do is click the qr code below to claim your offer!

REFERENCES

Body Fat Calculator & Body Fat Percentage Calculator. ACTIVE.com. Retrieved July 2020 Page url:https://www.active.com/fitness/calculators/bodyfat

Developing Explosive Strength and Power for Athletic Performance (2019). Jordan Syatt. Syatt Fitness. Retrieved July 2020 Page url: https://www.syattfitness.com/westside-barbell/developing-explosive-strength-and-power-for-athletic-performance/

Exercise and Type 2 Diabetes (2010). The American College of Sports Medicine and the American Diabetes Association: Joint position statement.PubMed Central (PMC). Retrieved July 2020 Page url: https://www.ncbi.nlm.nih.gov/pmc/articles/PMC2992225/

Five Benefits of Strength Training for Women (2019). YMCA. Retrieved July 2020 Page url: https://lafayettefamilyymca.org/five-benefits-of-strength-training-for-women/

How to use food to help your body fight inflammation (2019). Mayo Clinic. Retrieved July 2020 Page url: https://www.mayoclinic.org/healthy-

lifestyle/nutrition-and-healthy-eating/in-depth/how-to-use-food-to-help-your-body-fight-inflammation/art-20457586

Is Exercise a Viable Treatment for Depression. ACSMs Health Fit J. (2013). Duke University.PubMed Central. Retrieved July 2020 Page url: https://www.ncbi.nlm.nih.gov/pmc/articles/PMC3674785/

Older adults: Build Muscles and you'll live longer (2014). University of California – Los Angeles Health Sciences. ScienceDaily. Retrieved July 2020 Page url: https://www.sciencedaily.com/releases/2014/03/140314095102.htm

Resistance Training and Executive Functions: Improve focus (2010). PubMed Central. Retrieved July 2020 Page url: https://www.ncbi.nlm.nih.gov/pmc/articles/PMC3448565/

Resistance Training – Health benefits (2014). Department of Health& Human Services. Better Health Channel. Retrieved July 2020 Page url: https://www.betterhealth.vic.gov.au/health/healthyliving/resistance-training-health-benefits

Resistance Training For Children and Teens: Compelling Evidence of Benefits. Expert Group. MomsTeam. Retrieved July 2020 page url:- https://www.momsteam.com/health-safety/compelling-evidence-benefits-resistance-training-children-teens-experts-say

Strength Training in Children and Adolescents: Raising bar for Young Athletes (2009). PubMed Central (PMC). Retrieved July 2020 Page url: https://www.ncbi.nlm.nih.gov/pmc/articles/PMC3445252/

Training Power Systems: Anaerobic And Aerobic Training Methods! (2019). Rosie Chee. Retrieved July 2020 Page url: https://www.bodybuilding.com/fun/anaerobic-aerobic-training-methods.htm

Weightlifting is good for your heart and it doesn't take much (2018). Lowa

State University. News Service. Retrieved July 2020 Page url: https://www.news.iastate.edu/news/2018/11/13/resistancecvd

What is Cardiorespiratory Endurance and How Can You Improve It? (2013). Emily Cronkleton. Healthline. Retreived July 2020 Page url: https://www.healthline.com/health/cardiorespiratory-endurance

Wikipedia contributors (2020). Anaerobic exercise. Wikipedia. Retrieved July 2020 Page url:https://en.wikipedia.org/wiki/Anaerobic_exercise